# The Manual of
# Yoga
# Anatomy

# The Manual of
# Yoga
# Anatomy

Step-by-step guidance and anatomical analysis of **30 asanas**

QUAD BOOKS

Sally Parkes

Quarto is the authority on a wide range of topics.

Quarto educates, entertains and enriches the lives of our readers—enthusiasts and lovers of hands-on living.

www.QuartoKnows.com

First published in 2017 by

Global Book Publishing Pty Ltd

Part of The Quarto Group

Level One, Ovest House,

58 West Street, Brighton, BN1 2RA, UK

ISBN: 978-0-85762-518-2

A Global Book

Printed and Bound in China

Conceived, designed and produced by Global Book Publishing Pty Ltd

**Layout Design**:   Mike LeBihan
**Cover Design**:   Tony Seddon
**Cover Images**:   Joanna Culley, B.A. (Hons), R.M.I.P., M.M.M.A., medical-artist.com

**Illustrations** (Asanas): Joanna Culley, B.A., (Hons), R.M.I.P., M.M.M.A., medical-artist.com

**Illustrations** (Steps): Robert Brandt

**Additional Illustrations** (Anatomical):
David Carroll, Peter Child, Deborah Clarke, Geoff Cook, Marcus Cremonese, Beth Croce, Hans De Haas, Wendy de Paauw, Levant Efe, Mike Golding, Mike Gorman, Jeff Lang, Alex Lavroff, Ulrich Lehmann, Ruth Lindsay, Richard McKenna, Annabel Milne, Tony Pyrzakowski, Oliver Rennert, Caroline Rodrigues, Otto Schmidinger, Bob Seal, Vicky Short, Graeme Tavendale, Thomson Digital, Jonathan Tidball, Paul Tresnan, Valentin Varetsa, Glen Vause, Spike Wademan, Trevor Weekes, Paul Williams, David Wood

It is recommended that anyone who is considering participating in an exercise program should consult a physician before starting, and that no one should attempt a new exercise without the supervision of a qualified professional. While every care has been taken in presenting this material, the anatomical and medical information is not intended to replace professional medical advice. Neither the authors nor the publisher may be held responsible for any type of damage or harm caused by the misuse of information in this book.

# Contents

# How this Book Works

This book is organised into three primary sections: a full-colour anatomy overview; a principles of yoga section; and a full-colour illustrated guide to thirty yoga asana, comprising the main part of the book.

The Anatomy Overview section provides detailed, anatomically correct illustrations with clear, informative labels for the various body systems and regions.

The Principles of Yoga section examines the origins, history, and effects of the practice of yoga, and introduces some common yoga props and the four recurring starting positions that are referenced throughout the book.

The main content examining thirty yoga asanas is split into six chapters that divide the asanas into types – standing poses, standing balancing poses, standing forward bends, seated poses, backbending poses, and inversions.

Each yoga asana has four pages of explanation. The first two pages introduce the asana, summarise its benefits and origins, and offer tips on how to get the most out of it (while also advising what not to do). There are also clear step-by-step instructions and simple illustrations to help you achieve the correct posture.

The second two-page spread for each asana contains the more technical anatomical information – a brief summary discusses the main muscle activity in the asana, a clear table lists the main active muscles (and the type of activity), and stunning full-colour anatomical illustrations are labelled to show the key muscles used during the pose.

The book concludes with four pages of suggested sequences, allowing you to combine the asana into flowing movements.

## ANATOMY OVERVIEW PAGES

This section contains full-colour, double-page overview spreads that give a rundown of the important parts of a particular body system.

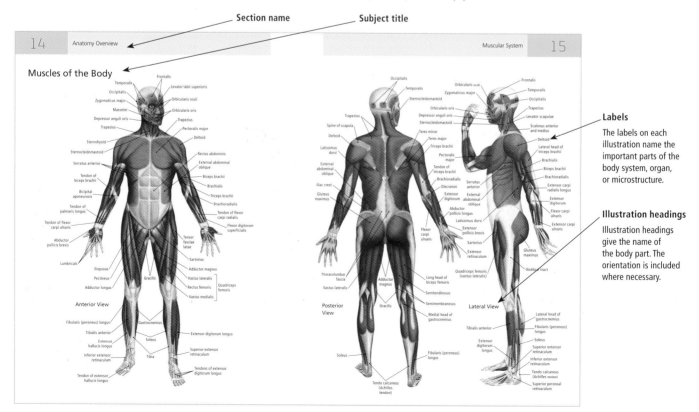

## ASANA STEP-BY-STEP PAGES

Chapter name — Asana name

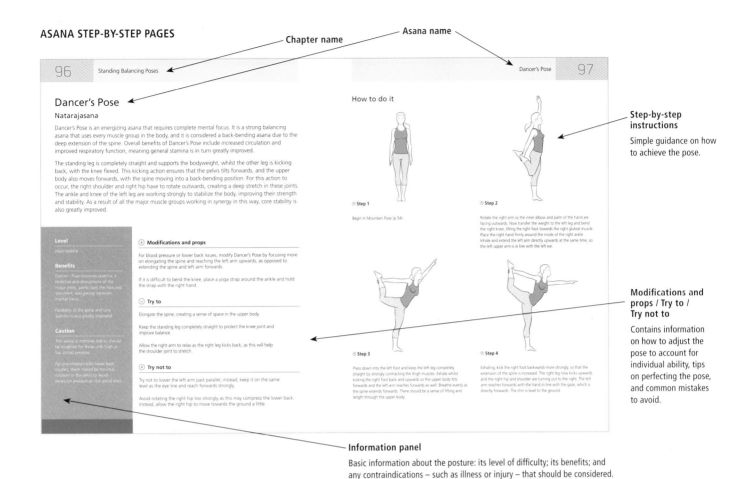

### Dancer's Pose
#### Natarajasana

Dancer's Pose is an energizing asana that requires complete mental focus. It is a strong balancing asana that uses every muscle group in the body, and it is considered a back-bending asana due to the deep extension of the spine. Overall benefits of Dancer's Pose include increased circulation and improved respiratory function, meaning general stamina is in turn greatly improved.

The standing leg is completely straight and supports the bodyweight, whilst the other leg is kicking back, with the knee flexed. This kicking action ensures that the pelvis tilts forwards, and the upper body also moves forwards, with the spine moving into a back-bending position. For this action to occur, the right shoulder and right hip have to rotate outwards, creating a deep stretch in these joints. The ankle and knee of the left leg are working strongly to stabilize the body, improving their strength and stability. As a result of all the major muscle groups working in synergy in this way, core stability is also greatly improved.

**Level**
Intermediate

**Benefits**
Dancer's Pose improves stamina, it stretches and strengthens all the major joints, particularly the hips and shoulders, and greatly improves mental focus.

Flexibility of the spine and core stability is also greatly improved.

**Caution**
This asana is intensive and so should be modified for those with high or low blood pressure.

For practitioners with lower back injuries, there should be minimal rotation in the pelvis to avoid excessive pressure on the spinal discs.

⊕ **Modifications and props**

For blood pressure or lower back issues, modify Dancer's Pose by focusing more on elongating the spine and reaching the left arm upwards, as opposed to extending the spine and left arm forwards.

If it is difficult to bend the knee, place a yoga strap around the ankle and hold the strap with the right hand.

⊘ **Try to**

Elongate the spine, creating a sense of space in the upper body.

Keep the standing leg completely straight to protect the knee joint and improve balance.

Allow the right arm to relax as the right leg kicks back, as this will help the shoulder joint to stretch.

⊘ **Try not to**

Try not to lower the left arm past parallel; instead, keep it on the same level as the eye line and reach forwards strongly.

Avoid rotating the right hip too strongly as this may compress the lower back. Instead, allow the right hip to move towards the ground a little.

**How to do it**

⊗ Step 1

Begin in Mountain Pose (p.54)

⊗ Step 2

Rotate the right arm so the inner elbow and palm of the hand are facing outwards. Now transfer the weight to the left leg and bend the right knee, lifting the right foot towards the right gluteal muscle. Place the right hand firmly around the inside of the right ankle. Inhale and extend the left arm directly upwards at the same time, so the left upper arm is in line with the left ear.

⊗ Step 3

Press down into the left foot and keep the left leg completely straight by strongly contracting the thigh muscles. Exhale whilst kicking the right foot back and upwards so the upper body tilts forwards and the left arm reaches forwards as well. Breathe evenly as the spine extends forwards. There should be a sense of lifting and length through the upper body.

⊗ Step 4

Exhaling, kick the right foot backwards more strongly, so that the extension of the spine is increased. The right leg now kicks upwards and the right hip and shoulder are turning out to the right. The left arm reaches forwards with the hand in line with the gaze, which is directly forwards. The chin is level to the ground.

**Step-by-step instructions**

Simple guidance on how to achieve the pose.

**Modifications and props / Try to / Try not to**

Contains information on how to adjust the pose to account for individual ability, tips on perfecting the pose, and common mistakes to avoid.

**Information panel**

Basic information about the posture: its level of difficulty; its benefits; and any contraindications – such as illness or injury – that should be considered.

## ASANA ANATOMY PAGES

### Dancer's Pose
#### Natarajasana

There are several muscle groups working differently during Dancer's Pose. The hamstrings of the right leg are shortening to create the flexion at the knee whilst the quadriceps and hip flexors are lengthening eccentrically. The posterior deltoid and rotator cuff of the right shoulder externally rotate the right arm. The triceps work concentrically to extend both arms, with the deltoid of the left shoulder contracting isometrically to hold the arm in place and the pectoral muscles working concentrically to assist. The left leg is fully extended with the quadriceps contracting concentrically and the hamstrings working to fixate this action. The pelvis is rotated anteriorly and the spine is extended in a back-bending position with the erector spinae shortening concentrically. The latissimus dorsi and rectus abdominis help to fixate the position of the spine.

**muscle activity**

**prime mover**
1  Quadriceps
2  Hamstrings
3  Erector spinae
4  Deltoids
5  Gluteus minimus and maximus

**antagonist**
6  Rectus abdominis
7  Pectoralis major and minor
8  Latissimus dorsi

(3 beneath thoracolumbar fascia)

**spine**
The spine is in extension, moving in a sagittal plane from a frontal axis.
The pelvis is in an anterior tilt position.

**Anatomy of the pose**

4  Deltoids

Latissimus dorsi

Pectoralis major and minor

Quadriceps 1

Rectus abdominis

Gluteus minimus and maximus

Hamstrings 2

Not visible from this view:
3  Erector spinae (on back)

**Illustrations**

Full-colour anatomical illustrations show the superficial musculature during each pose.

**Labels**

Identify the location of the muscles discussed (brackets indicate where deeper muscles are not visible). Prime movers are identified with a yellow dot, antagonists with blue.

**Muscle information**

Lists the main muscles for the pose, identifying prime movers and antagonists, and shows muscle location on front and back view figure.

# Anatomy Overview

# Body Regions

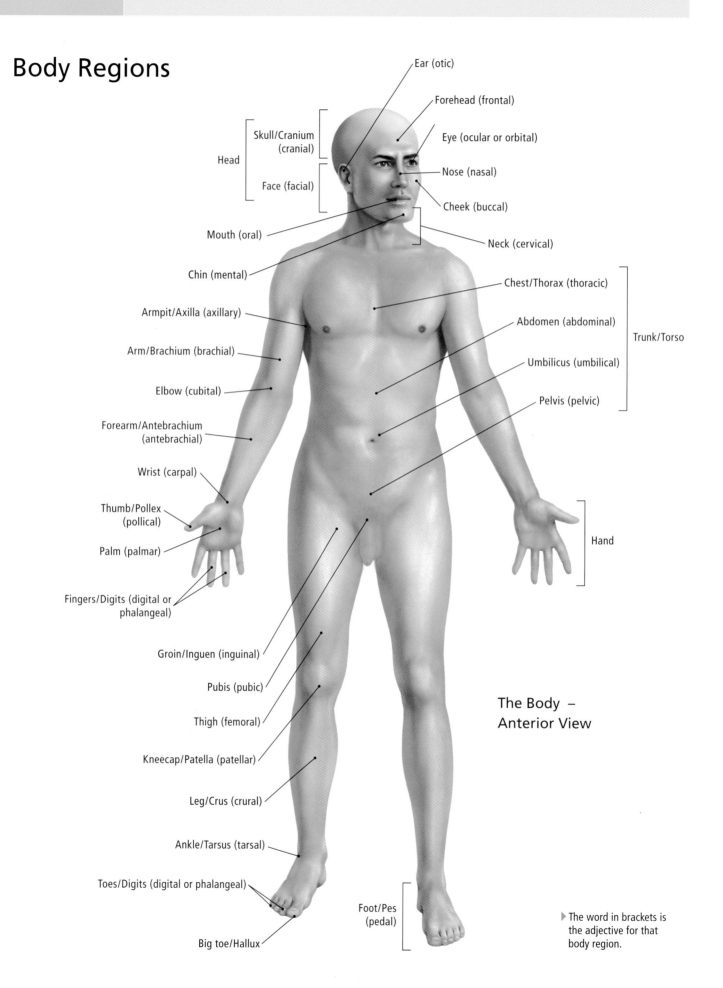

Ear (otic)

Forehead (frontal)

Skull/Cranium (cranial)

Head

Eye (ocular or orbital)

Face (facial)

Nose (nasal)

Cheek (buccal)

Mouth (oral)

Neck (cervical)

Chin (mental)

Chest/Thorax (thoracic)

Armpit/Axilla (axillary)

Abdomen (abdominal)

Arm/Brachium (brachial)

Trunk/Torso

Umbilicus (umbilical)

Elbow (cubital)

Pelvis (pelvic)

Forearm/Antebrachium (antebrachial)

Wrist (carpal)

Thumb/Pollex (pollical)

Hand

Palm (palmar)

Fingers/Digits (digital or phalangeal)

Groin/Inguen (inguinal)

Pubis (pubic)

The Body –
Anterior View

Thigh (femoral)

Kneecap/Patella (patellar)

Leg/Crus (crural)

Ankle/Tarsus (tarsal)

Toes/Digits (digital or phalangeal)

Foot/Pes (pedal)

▶ The word in brackets is the adjective for that body region.

Big toe/Hallux

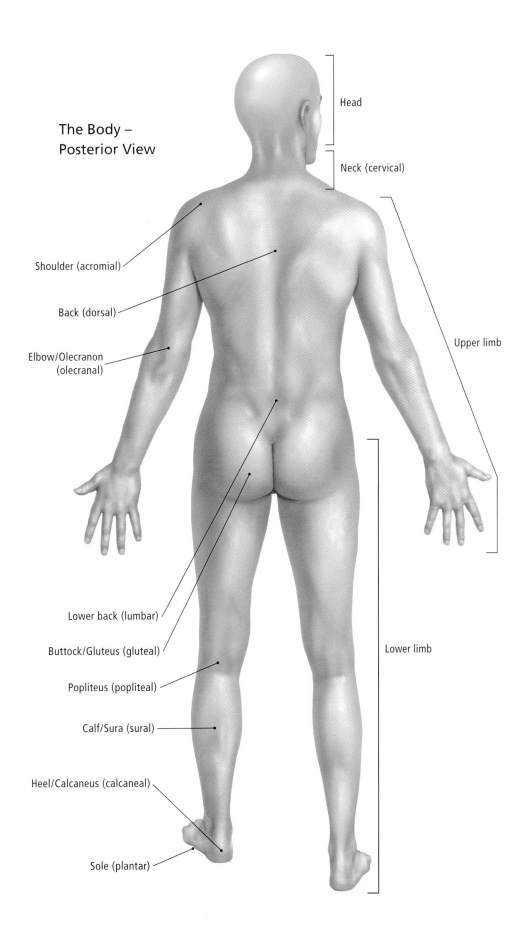

The Body –
Posterior View

Head

Neck (cervical)

Shoulder (acromial)

Back (dorsal)

Elbow/Olecranon
(olecranal)

Upper limb

Lower back (lumbar)

Buttock/Gluteus (gluteal)

Popliteus (popliteal)

Lower limb

Calf/Sura (sural)

Heel/Calcaneus (calcaneal)

Sole (plantar)

# Muscles of the Body

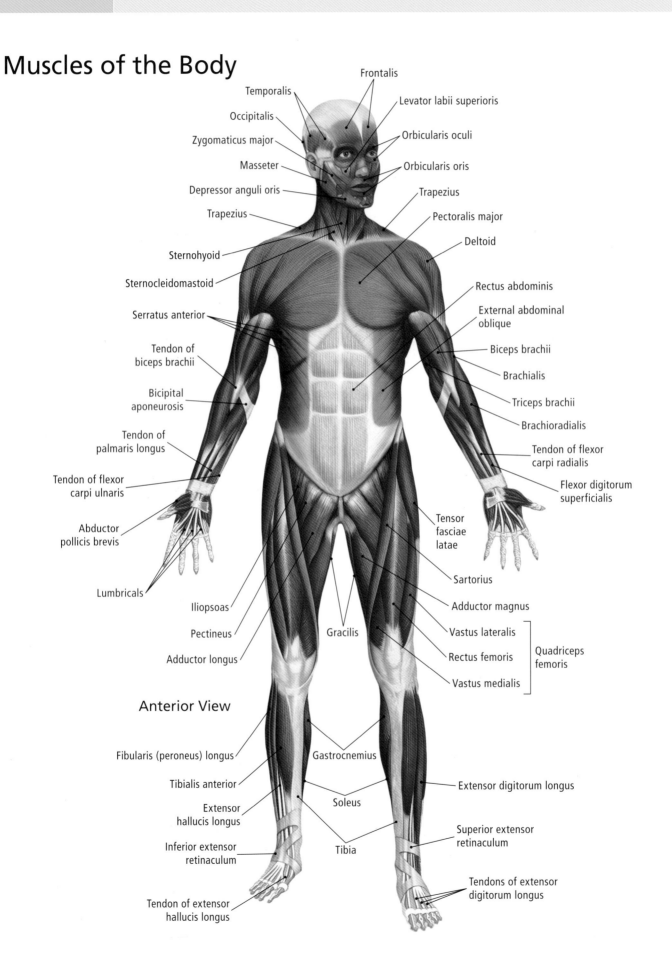

Frontalis

Temporalis

Levator labii superioris

Occipitalis

Zygomaticus major

Orbicularis oculi

Masseter

Orbicularis oris

Depressor anguli oris

Trapezius

Trapezius

Pectoralis major

Sternohyoid

Deltoid

Sternocleidomastoid

Rectus abdominis

Serratus anterior

External abdominal oblique

Tendon of biceps brachii

Biceps brachii

Bicipital aponeurosis

Brachialis

Triceps brachii

Tendon of palmaris longus

Brachioradialis

Tendon of flexor carpi ulnaris

Tendon of flexor carpi radialis

Abductor pollicis brevis

Flexor digitorum superficialis

Tensor fasciae latae

Lumbricals

Sartorius

Iliopsoas

Adductor magnus

Pectineus

Gracilis

Vastus lateralis

Adductor longus

Rectus femoris

Quadriceps femoris

Vastus medialis

**Anterior View**

Fibularis (peroneus) longus

Gastrocnemius

Tibialis anterior

Extensor digitorum longus

Extensor hallucis longus

Soleus

Inferior extensor retinaculum

Superior extensor retinaculum

Tibia

Tendon of extensor hallucis longus

Tendons of extensor digitorum longus

Occipitalis

Temporalis

Sternocleidomastoid

Trapezius

Spine of scapula

Deltoid

Latissimus dorsi

External abdominal oblique

Iliac crest

Gluteus maximus

Thoracolumbar fascia

Vastus lateralis

**Posterior View**

Teres minor

Teres major

Triceps brachii

Pectoralis major

Tendon of triceps brachii

Brachioradialis

Olecranon

Extensor digitorum

Abductor pollicis longus

Extensor pollicis brevis

Flexor carpi ulnaris

Extensor retinaculum

Adductor magnus

Gracilis

Long head of biceps femoris

Semitendinosus

Semimembranosus

Medial head of gastrocnemius

Fibularis (peroneus) longus

Soleus

Tendo calcaneus (Achilles tendon)

Orbicularis oculi

Zygomaticus major

Orbicularis oris

Depressor anguli oris

Sternocleidomastoid

Serratus anterior

External abdominal oblique

Latissimus dorsi

Sartorius

Quadriceps femoris (vastus lateralis)

Frontalis

Temporalis

Occipitalis

Trapezius

Levator scapulae

Scalenus anterior and medius

Deltoid

Lateral head of triceps brachii

Brachialis

Biceps brachii

Brachioradialis

Extensor carpi radialis longus

Extensor digitorum

Flexor carpi ulnaris

Extensor carpi ulnaris

Gluteus maximus

Iliotibial tract

**Lateral View**

Tibialis anterior

Extensor digitorum longus

Lateral head of gastrocnemius

Fibularis (peroneus) longus

Soleus

Superior extensor retinaculum

Inferior extensor retinaculum

Tendo calcaneus (Achilles tendon)

Superior peroneal retinaculum

# Muscles of the Abdomen and Back

Muscles of the Abdomen –
Anterior View

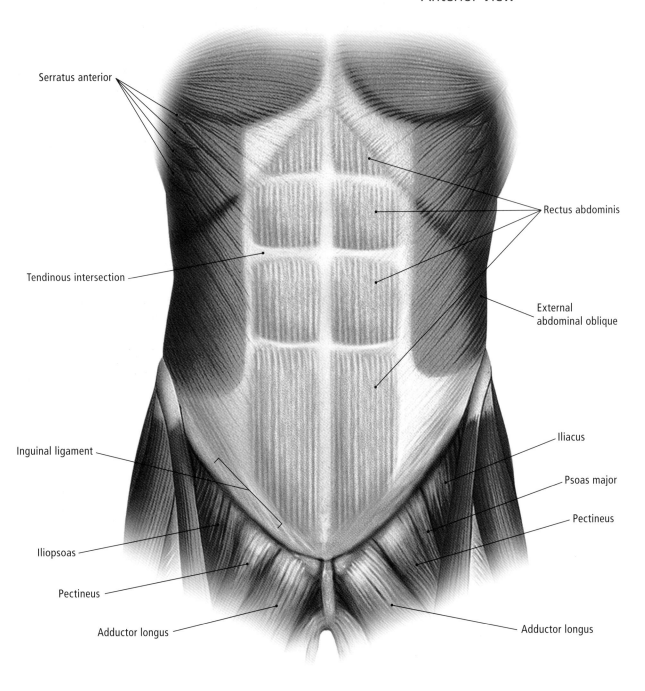

Serratus anterior

Tendinous intersection

Inguinal ligament

Iliopsoas

Pectineus

Adductor longus

Rectus abdominis

External
abdominal oblique

Iliacus

Psoas major

Pectineus

Adductor longus

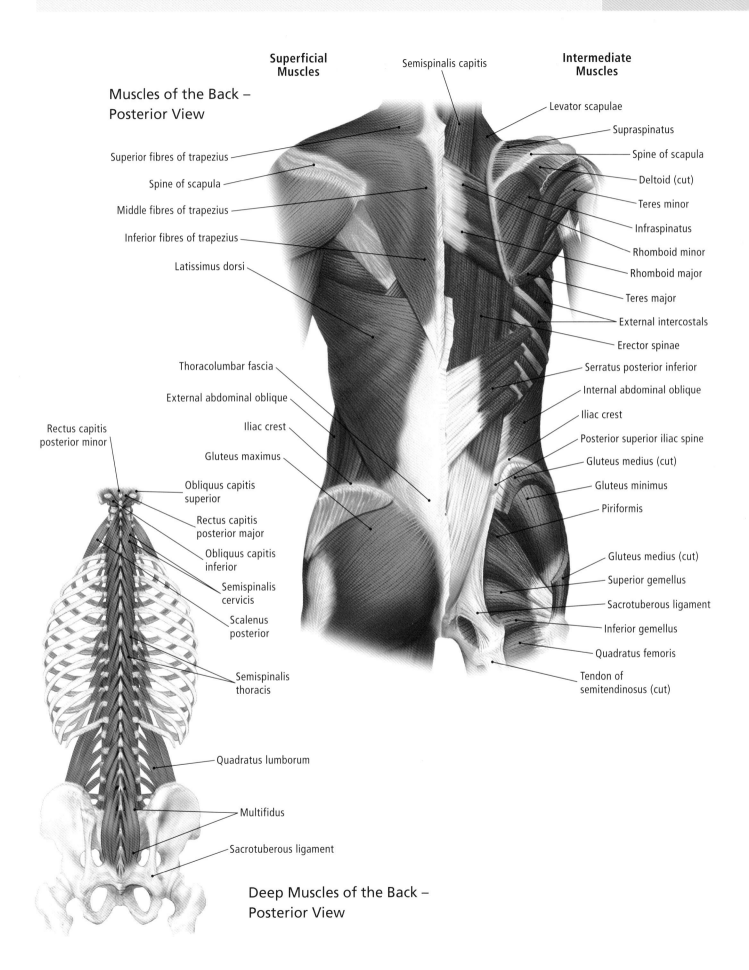

**Superficial Muscles**

Semispinalis capitis

**Intermediate Muscles**

### Muscles of the Back – Posterior View

Superior fibres of trapezius

Spine of scapula

Middle fibres of trapezius

Inferior fibres of trapezius

Latissimus dorsi

Thoracolumbar fascia

External abdominal oblique

Iliac crest

Gluteus maximus

Rectus capitis posterior minor

Obliquus capitis superior

Rectus capitis posterior major

Obliquus capitis inferior

Semispinalis cervicis

Scalenus posterior

Semispinalis thoracis

Levator scapulae

Supraspinatus

Spine of scapula

Deltoid (cut)

Teres minor

Infraspinatus

Rhomboid minor

Rhomboid major

Teres major

External intercostals

Erector spinae

Serratus posterior inferior

Internal abdominal oblique

Iliac crest

Posterior superior iliac spine

Gluteus medius (cut)

Gluteus minimus

Piriformis

Gluteus medius (cut)

Superior gemellus

Sacrotuberous ligament

Inferior gemellus

Quadratus femoris

Tendon of semitendinosus (cut)

Quadratus lumborum

Multifidus

Sacrotuberous ligament

### Deep Muscles of the Back – Posterior View

# Muscles of the Upper and Lower Limb

Pectoralis major

Spine of scapula

Deltoid

**Superficial Muscles of the Upper Limb – Posterior View**

Deltoid

Biceps brachii

Brachialis

Long head of triceps brachii

Lateral head of triceps brachii

Tendon of triceps brachii

Brachioradialis

Triceps brachii

Pronator teres

Brachioradialis

Anconeus

Olecranon

Extensor digiti minimi

Tendon of flexor carpi radialis

Tendon of palmaris longus

Flexor carpi ulnaris

Extensor digitorum

Tendon of flexor carpi ulnaris

Abductor pollicis longus

Flexor digitorum superficialis

Flexor retinaculum

Extensor pollicis brevis

Palmaris brevis

Extensor retinaculum

Hypothenar muscles

Thenar muscles

**Superficial Muscles of the Upper Limb – Anterior View**

Fibrous flexor sheath

Tendons of extensors of the digits

Inguinal ligament

Iliopsoas

Pectineus

Adductor longus

Gracilis

Iliotibial tract

Fibularis (peroneus) longus

Extensor digitorum longus

Tibialis anterior

Superior extensor retinaculum

Inferior extensor retinaculum

Gastrocnemius

Soleus

**Superficial Muscles of the Lower Limb – Anterior View**

Gluteus medius

Gluteus maximus

Iliotibial tract

Biceps femoris

Adductor magnus

Semimembranosus

Semitendinosus

Gracilis

Lateral head of gastrocnemius

Medial head of gastrocnemius

**Superficial Muscles of the Lower Limb – Posterior View**

# Bones of the Body

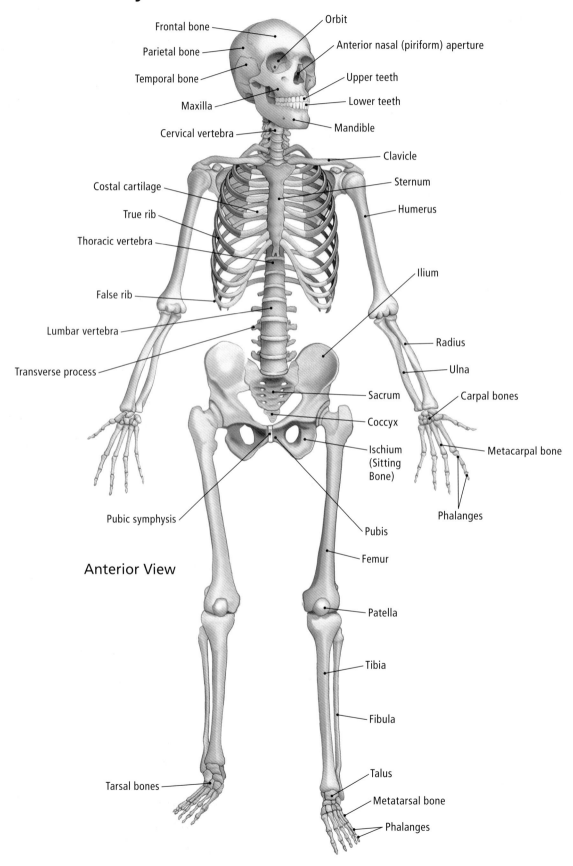

Frontal bone

Parietal bone

Temporal bone

Maxilla

Cervical vertebra

Costal cartilage

True rib

Thoracic vertebra

False rib

Lumbar vertebra

Transverse process

Pubic symphysis

Anterior View

Orbit

Anterior nasal (piriform) aperture

Upper teeth

Lower teeth

Mandible

Clavicle

Sternum

Humerus

Ilium

Radius

Ulna

Carpal bones

Metacarpal bone

Phalanges

Sacrum

Coccyx

Ischium (Sitting Bone)

Pubis

Femur

Patella

Tibia

Fibula

Talus

Metatarsal bone

Phalanges

Tarsal bones

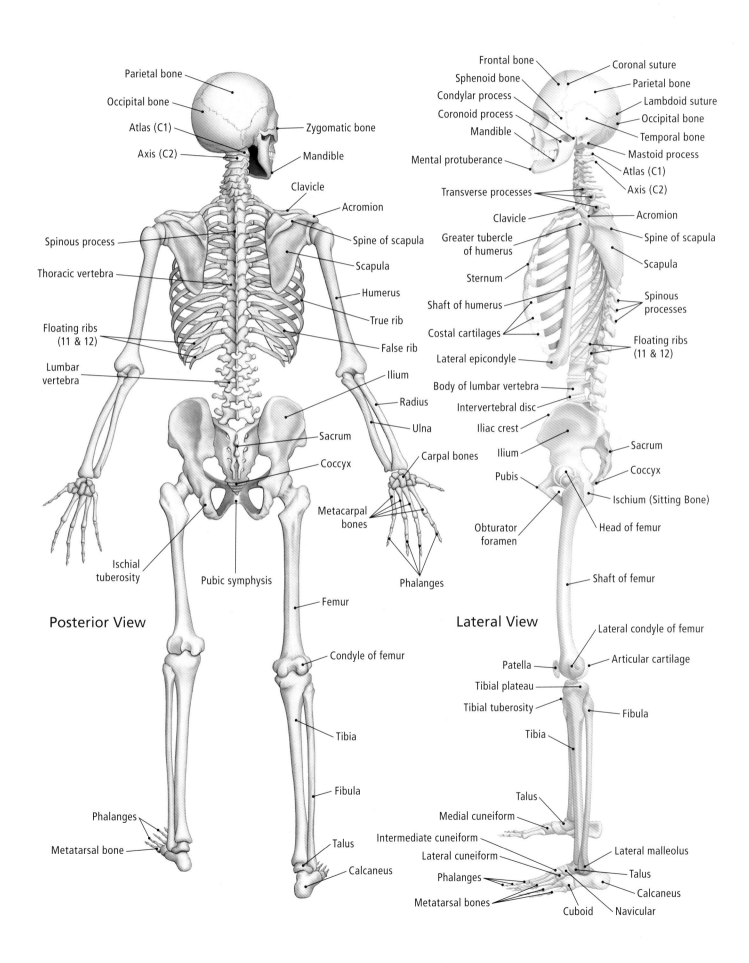

**Posterior View**

- Parietal bone
- Occipital bone
- Atlas (C1)
- Axis (C2)
- Zygomatic bone
- Mandible
- Clavicle
- Acromion
- Spine of scapula
- Scapula
- Humerus
- True rib
- Spinous process
- Thoracic vertebra
- Floating ribs (11 & 12)
- False rib
- Lumbar vertebra
- Ilium
- Radius
- Ulna
- Sacrum
- Coccyx
- Carpal bones
- Metacarpal bones
- Ischial tuberosity
- Pubic symphysis
- Phalanges
- Femur
- Condyle of femur
- Tibia
- Fibula
- Phalanges
- Metatarsal bone
- Talus
- Calcaneus

**Lateral View**

- Frontal bone
- Sphenoid bone
- Condylar process
- Coronoid process
- Mandible
- Mental protuberance
- Coronal suture
- Parietal bone
- Lambdoid suture
- Occipital bone
- Temporal bone
- Mastoid process
- Atlas (C1)
- Axis (C2)
- Transverse processes
- Clavicle
- Greater tubercle of humerus
- Sternum
- Shaft of humerus
- Costal cartilages
- Lateral epicondyle
- Body of lumbar vertebra
- Intervertebral disc
- Iliac crest
- Ilium
- Pubis
- Obturator foramen
- Acromion
- Spine of scapula
- Scapula
- Spinous processes
- Floating ribs (11 & 12)
- Sacrum
- Coccyx
- Ischium (Sitting Bone)
- Head of femur
- Shaft of femur
- Lateral condyle of femur
- Articular cartilage
- Patella
- Tibial plateau
- Tibial tuberosity
- Fibula
- Tibia
- Talus
- Medial cuneiform
- Intermediate cuneiform
- Lateral cuneiform
- Phalanges
- Metatarsal bones
- Lateral malleolus
- Talus
- Calcaneus
- Cuboid
- Navicular

# Vertebral Column

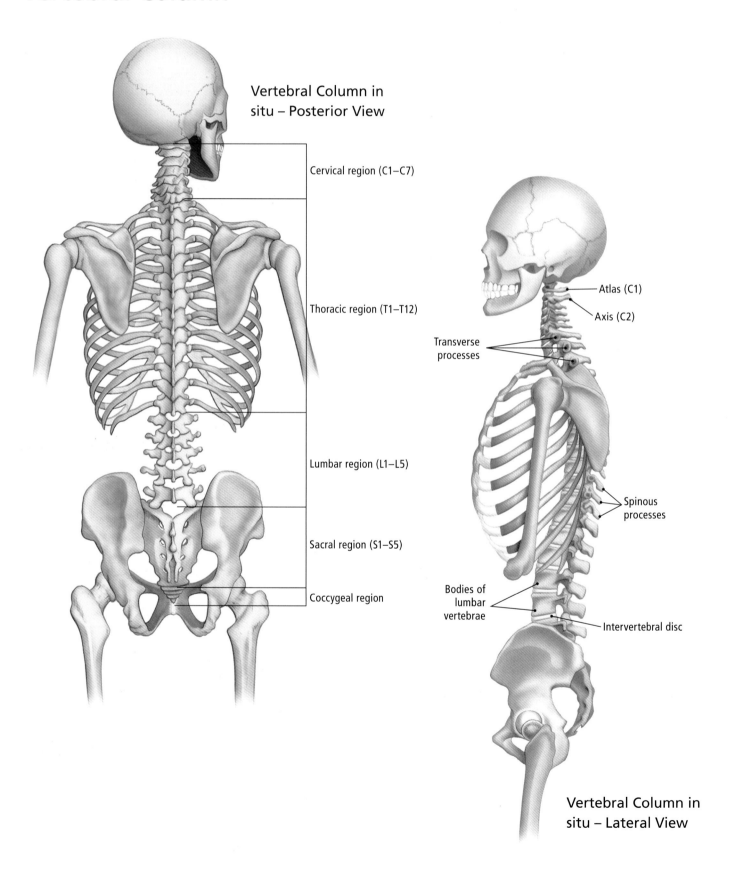

Vertebral Column in
situ – Posterior View

Cervical region (C1–C7)

Thoracic region (T1–T12)

Lumbar region (L1–L5)

Sacral region (S1–S5)

Coccygeal region

Atlas (C1)

Axis (C2)

Transverse
processes

Spinous
processes

Bodies of
lumbar
vertebrae

Intervertebral disc

Vertebral Column in
situ – Lateral View

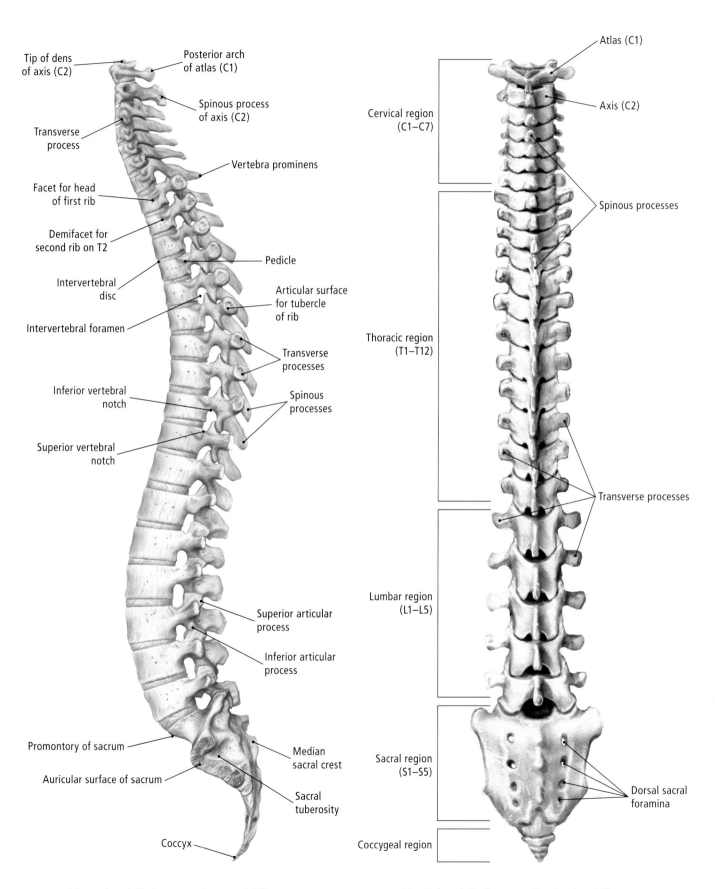

Tip of dens of axis (C2)

Posterior arch of atlas (C1)

Spinous process of axis (C2)

Transverse process

Vertebra prominens

Facet for head of first rib

Demifacet for second rib on T2

Pedicle

Intervertebral disc

Articular surface for tubercle of rib

Intervertebral foramen

Transverse processes

Inferior vertebral notch

Spinous processes

Superior vertebral notch

Superior articular process

Inferior articular process

Promontory of sacrum

Auricular surface of sacrum

Median sacral crest

Sacral tuberosity

Coccyx

Atlas (C1)

Axis (C2)

Cervical region (C1–C7)

Spinous processes

Thoracic region (T1–T12)

Transverse processes

Lumbar region (L1–L5)

Sacral region (S1–S5)

Dorsal sacral foramina

Coccygeal region

**Vertebral Column – Lateral View**

**Vertebral Column – Posterior View**

# Bones of the Upper and Lower Limb

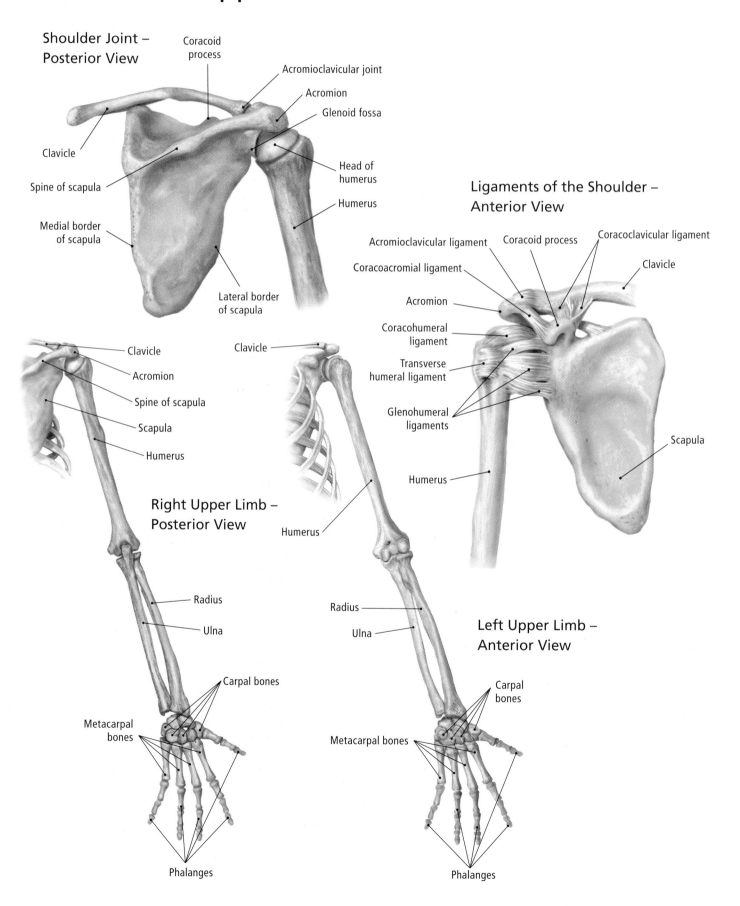

Shoulder Joint – Posterior View

Coracoid process

Acromioclavicular joint

Acromion

Glenoid fossa

Clavicle

Head of humerus

Spine of scapula

Humerus

Medial border of scapula

Lateral border of scapula

Ligaments of the Shoulder – Anterior View

Acromioclavicular ligament

Coracoid process

Coracoclavicular ligament

Coracoacromial ligament

Clavicle

Acromion

Coracohumeral ligament

Transverse humeral ligament

Glenohumeral ligaments

Scapula

Humerus

Clavicle

Acromion

Spine of scapula

Scapula

Humerus

Right Upper Limb – Posterior View

Clavicle

Humerus

Radius

Ulna

Radius

Ulna

Left Upper Limb – Anterior View

Carpal bones

Carpal bones

Metacarpal bones

Metacarpal bones

Phalanges

Phalanges

## Right Lower Limb – Anterior View

## Left Lower Limb – Posterior View

Femur

Patella

Tibia

Fibula

Talus

Tarsal bones

Metatarsal bones

Phalanges

Calcaneus

## Bones and Ligaments of the Knee – Anterior View

Femur

Lateral condyle of femur

Fibular (lateral) collateral ligament

Lateral meniscus

Posterior cruciate ligament

Anterior cruciate ligament

Medial condyle of femur

Medial meniscus

Tibial (medial) collateral ligament

Patellar ligament

Patella

Tibia

## Ligaments of the Ankle and Foot – Lateral View

Fibula

Tibia

Anterior tibiofibular ligament

Posterior tibiofibular ligament

Calcaneofibular ligament

Anterior talofibular ligament

Dorsal cuboideonavicular ligament

Dorsal cuneonavicular ligaments

Dorsal intercuneiform ligament

Dorsal tarsometatarsal ligaments

Calcaneus

Talocalcaneal ligaments

Bifurcate ligament

Dorsal calcaneocuboid ligament

Dorsal cuneocuboid ligament

Dorsal metatarsal ligaments

# Nervous System

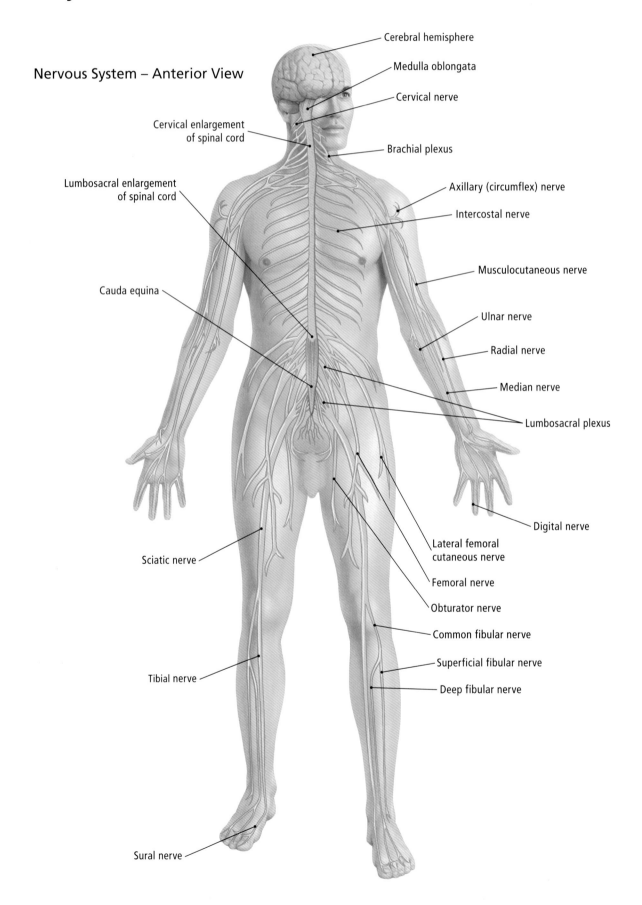

Nervous System – Anterior View

Cerebral hemisphere

Medulla oblongata

Cervical nerve

Cervical enlargement of spinal cord

Brachial plexus

Lumbosacral enlargement of spinal cord

Axillary (circumflex) nerve

Intercostal nerve

Musculocutaneous nerve

Cauda equina

Ulnar nerve

Radial nerve

Median nerve

Lumbosacral plexus

Digital nerve

Sciatic nerve

Lateral femoral cutaneous nerve

Femoral nerve

Obturator nerve

Common fibular nerve

Superficial fibular nerve

Tibial nerve

Deep fibular nerve

Sural nerve

## Central Nervous System

Cerebrum

Pons

Cerebellum

Spinal cord

Conus medullaris

Cauda equina

## Autonomic Nervous System

Parasympathetic division

Spinal cord

Sympathetic division

Parasympathetic division

Sacrum

# Spinal Cord

## Spinal Cord – Cross-sectional View

Lateral corticospinal tract
Dorsal funiculus
Central canal
Spinal grey matter
Gracile fasciculus
Lateral funiculus
Lateral reticulospinal tract
Cuneate fasciculus
Lateral vestibulospinal tract
Dorsolateral sulcus
Medial reticulospinal tract
Dorsal spino-cerebellar tract
Medial vestibulospinal tract
Anterior corticospinal tract
Spinothalamic tract
Ventral funiculus
Ventral spinocerebellar tract
Anterior median fissure
Posterior radicular artery
Dorsal horn
Anterior radicular vein
Posterior spinal vein
Central canal
Spinal (dorsal root) ganglion
Posterior spinal artery
Anterior ramus of spinal nerve
Ventral horn
Dorsal rootlets
Sulcal vein
Posterior radicular artery
Anterior radicular artery
Spinal (dorsal root) ganglion
Epineurium
Posterior ramus of spinal nerve
Perineurium
Anterior ramus of spinal nerve
Grey ramus communicans
Endoneurium
White ramus communicans
Ventral rootlets
Ventral rootlets
Pia mater
Node of Ranvier
Axon
Dura mater
Anterior spinal vein
Anterior spinal artery
Arachnoid
Myelin sheath of Schwann cell

## Spinal Nerves

## Spinal Cord – Anterior View

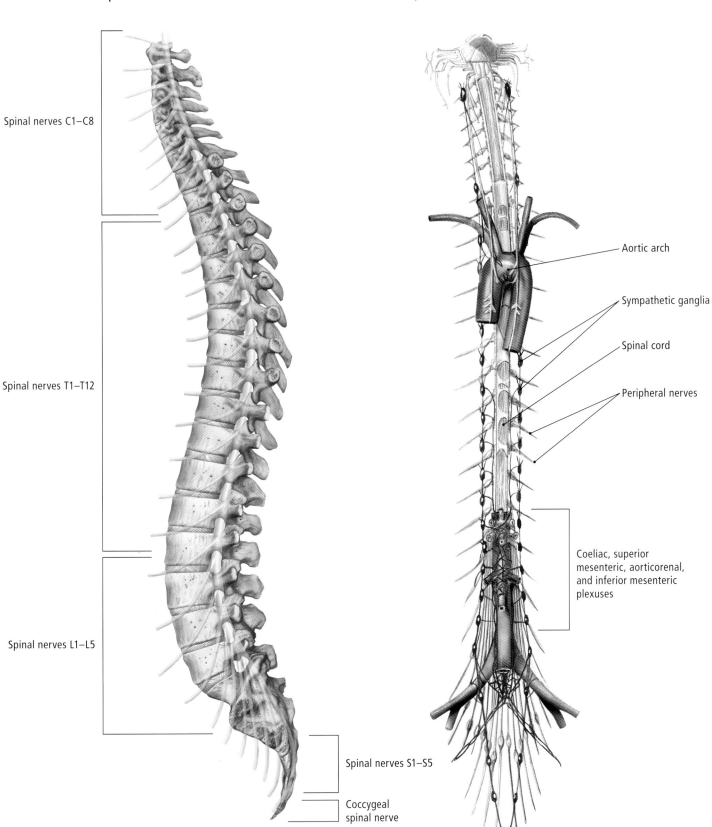

Spinal nerves C1–C8

Spinal nerves T1–T12

Spinal nerves L1–L5

Spinal nerves S1–S5

Coccygeal
spinal nerve

Aortic arch

Sympathetic ganglia

Spinal cord

Peripheral nerves

Coeliac, superior
mesenteric, aorticorenal,
and inferior mesenteric
plexuses

# Circulatory System

Superficial temporal vein
Posterior auricular vein
External jugular vein
Internal jugular vein
Brachiocephalic vein
Subclavian vein
Superior vena cava
Axillary vein
Cephalic vein
Brachial vein
Basilic vein
Azygos vein
Median cubital vein
Renal vein
Inferior vena cava
Radial vein
Ulnar vein
Common iliac vein
Palmar venous arch
Digital veins

Superficial temporal artery
Posterior auricular artery
Facial artery
Common carotid artery
Subclavian artery
Axillary artery
Aortic arch
Intercostal arteries
Brachial artery
Descending aorta
Renal artery
Superior ulnar collateral artery
Common iliac artery
Ulnar artery
Radial artery
Deep palmar arterial arch
Digital arteries
External iliac artery
Internal iliac artery
Deep femoral artery
Femoral artery
Popliteal artery
Fibular artery
Anterior tibial artery
Posterior tibial artery

External iliac vein
Internal iliac vein
Femoral vein
Great saphenous vein
Popliteal vein
Small saphenous vein
Fibular vein
Anterior tibial vein

Dorsalis pedis artery
Dorsal arch
Plantar arch
Digital arteries

Dorsal venous arch
Plantar venous arch
Digital veins

## Circulatory System – Anterior View

**Heart – Anterior View**

- Brachiocephalic artery (trunk)
- Left common carotid artery
- Right brachiocephalic vein
- Left subclavian artery
- Left brachiocephalic vein
- Superior vena cava
- Aortic arch
- Right atrium
- Ligamentum arteriosum
- Right pulmonary artery
- Left pulmonary artery
- Left superior pulmonary vein
- Right superior pulmonary vein
- Left inferior pulmonary vein
- Right inferior pulmonary vein
- Left atrium
- Right coronary artery
- Diagonal branch
- Anterior descending branch of left coronary artery
- Right marginal branch of right coronary artery
- Left ventricle
- Right ventricle
- Inferior vena cava
- Descending aorta

**Heart – Posterior View**

- Left common carotid artery
- Left subclavian artery
- Brachiocephalic artery (trunk)
- Aortic arch
- Superior vena cava
- Left pulmonary artery
- Pericardium
- Pericardium
- Right superior pulmonary vein
- Right pulmonary artery
- Right inferior pulmonary vein
- Left superior pulmonary vein
- Right atrium
- Left inferior pulmonary vein
- Inferior vena cava
- Posterior ventricular branch of left coronary artery
- Right coronary artery
- Left ventricle
- Posterior descending branch of right coronary artery
- Right ventricle

# Blood Vessels of the Upper and Lower Limb

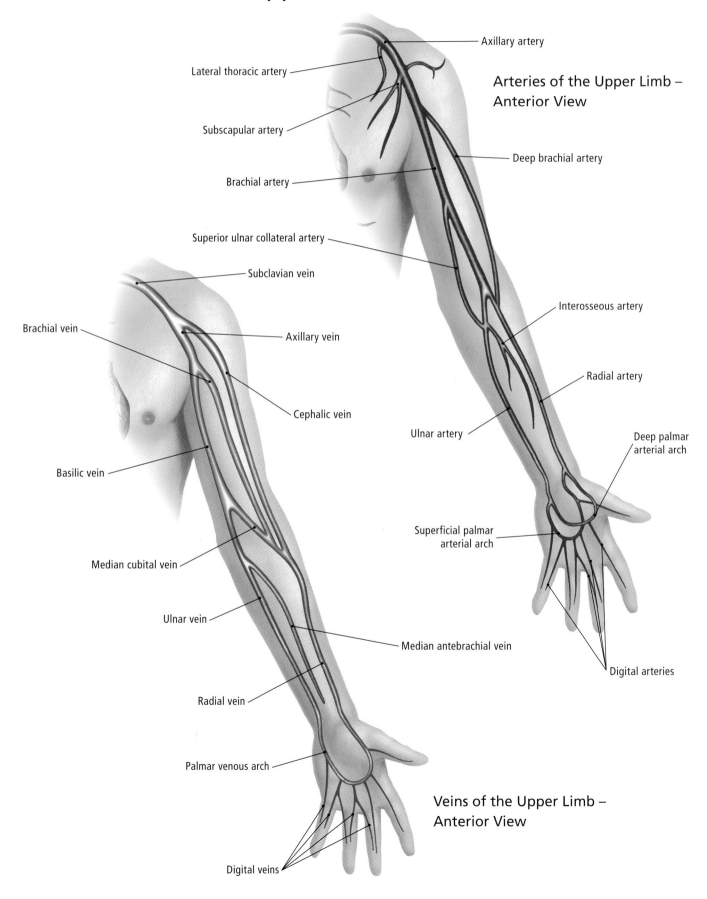

Lateral thoracic artery

Subscapular artery

Brachial artery

Superior ulnar collateral artery

Subclavian vein

Brachial vein

Basilic vein

Median cubital vein

Ulnar vein

Radial vein

Palmar venous arch

Digital veins

Axillary artery

Arteries of the Upper Limb –
Anterior View

Deep brachial artery

Interosseous artery

Radial artery

Deep palmar
arterial arch

Ulnar artery

Superficial palmar
arterial arch

Digital arteries

Axillary vein

Cephalic vein

Median antebrachial vein

Veins of the Upper Limb –
Anterior View

Arteries of the Lower Limb –
Anterior View

External iliac artery

Deep femoral artery

Femoral artery

Obturator artery

Popliteal artery

Descending
genicular artery

Posterior tibial artery

Fibular artery

Anterior tibial artery

Dorsalis pedis artery

Digital arteries

Dorsal arch

Plantar arch

External iliac vein

Obturator vein

Femoral vein

Popliteal vein

Great saphenous
vein

Small saphenous vein

Anterior tibial vein

Fibular vein

Posterior tibial vein

Digital veins

Dorsal venous arch

Plantar venous arch

Veins of the Lower Limb
– Anterior View

# Respiratory System

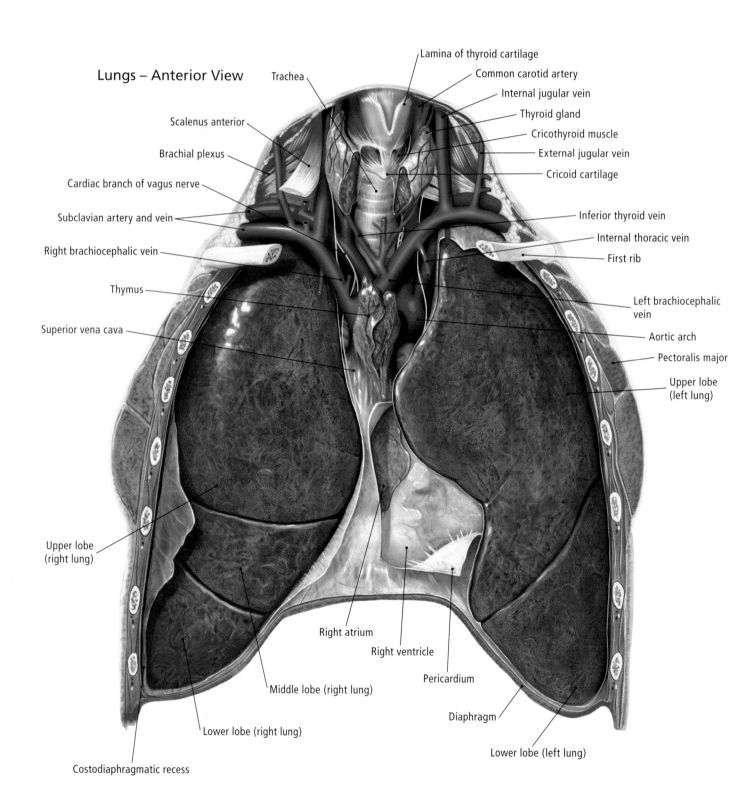

Lungs – Anterior View

Trachea

Lamina of thyroid cartilage

Common carotid artery

Internal jugular vein

Thyroid gland

Cricothyroid muscle

External jugular vein

Cricoid cartilage

Scalenus anterior

Brachial plexus

Cardiac branch of vagus nerve

Subclavian artery and vein

Inferior thyroid vein

Internal thoracic vein

First rib

Right brachiocephalic vein

Thymus

Left brachiocephalic vein

Superior vena cava

Aortic arch

Pectoralis major

Upper lobe (left lung)

Upper lobe (right lung)

Right atrium

Right ventricle

Pericardium

Diaphragm

Middle lobe (right lung)

Lower lobe (right lung)

Lower lobe (left lung)

Costodiaphragmatic recess

## Respiratory System – Anterior View

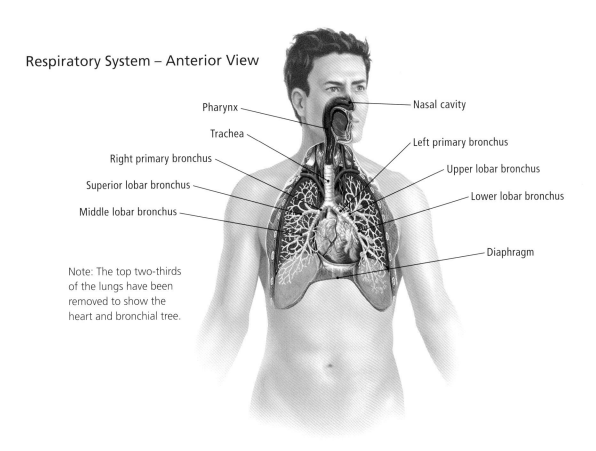

Pharynx

Nasal cavity

Trachea

Left primary bronchus

Right primary bronchus

Upper lobar bronchus

Superior lobar bronchus

Lower lobar bronchus

Middle lobar bronchus

Diaphragm

Note: The top two-thirds
of the lungs have been
removed to show the
heart and bronchial tree.

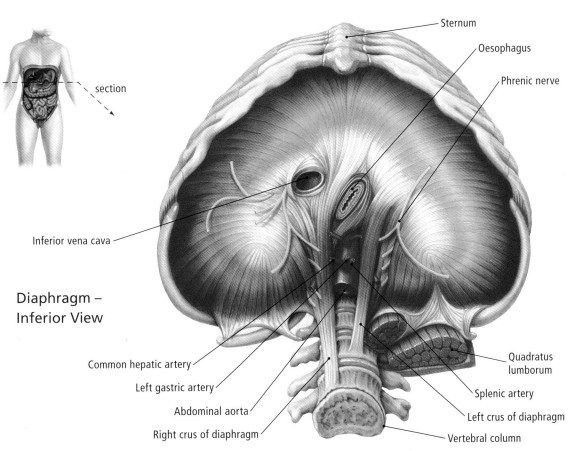

section

## Diaphragm – Inferior View

Sternum

Oesophagus

Phrenic nerve

Inferior vena cava

Common hepatic artery

Quadratus
lumborum

Left gastric artery

Splenic artery

Abdominal aorta

Left crus of diaphragm

Right crus of diaphragm

Vertebral column

# Movements of the Body

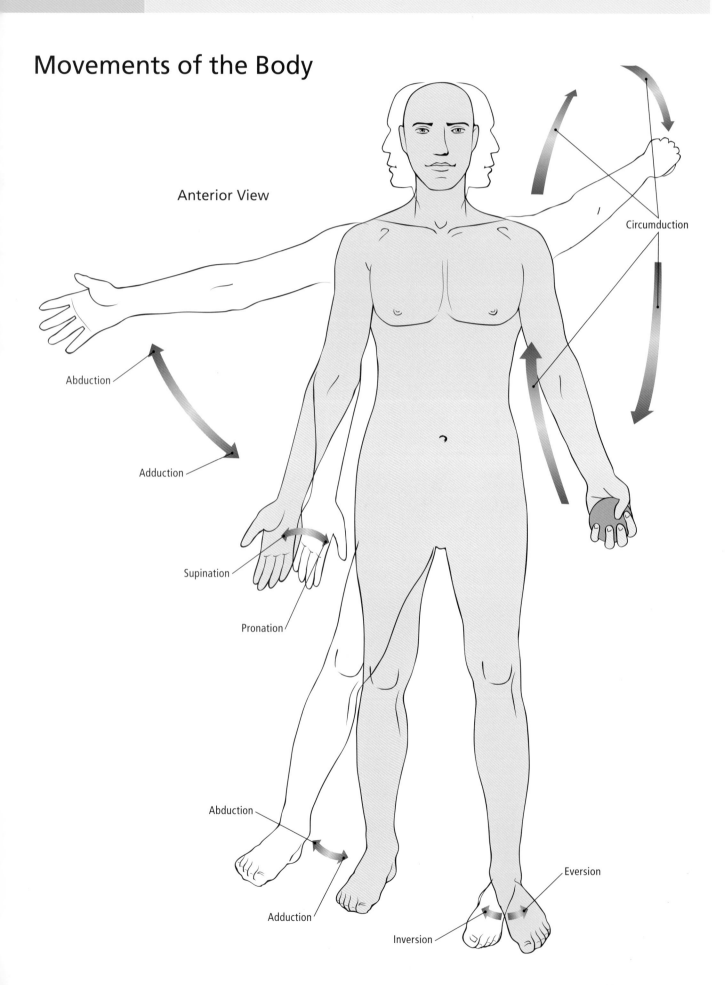

Anterior View

Abduction

Adduction

Supination

Pronation

Circumduction

Abduction

Adduction

Eversion

Inversion

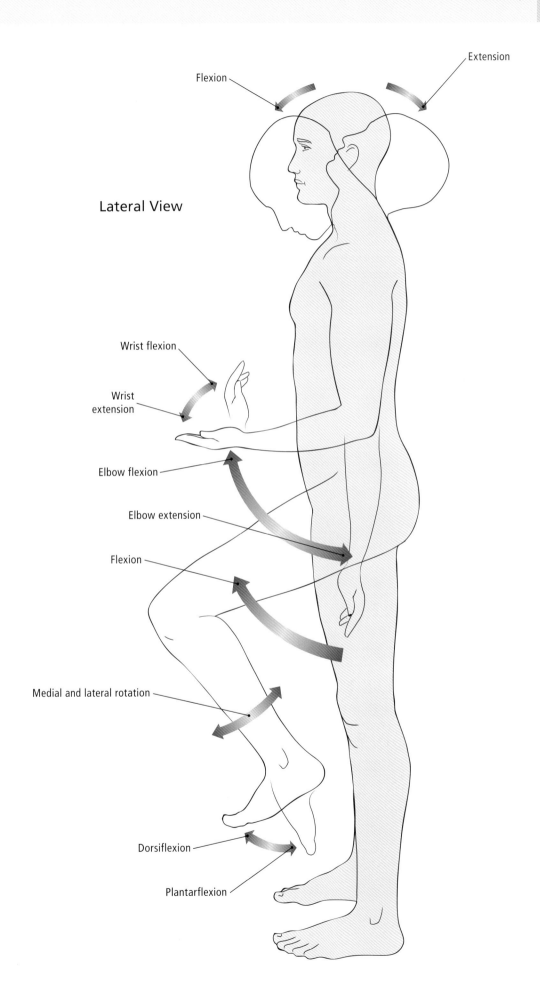

Flexion

Extension

Lateral View

Wrist flexion

Wrist extension

Elbow flexion

Elbow extension

Flexion

Medial and lateral rotation

Dorsiflexion

Plantarflexion

# Principles of Yoga

Yoga is an approach to life that helps us on the path to a more healthy and content way of being. It is an ancient system that intertwines many physical and spiritual practices which are designed not only to develop the body, but to broaden our mental faculties and spiritual capacities. The principles practised within this system include focused breathing, meditation, relaxation, and a healthy diet, and, of course, exercise in the form of asanas, or postures, the practice of which makes up the main content of this book.

# What Is Yoga?

The word 'yoga' comes from the Sanskrit word for root, *yuj*, which in this context means 'to join', 'to yoke', or 'to unite' – the union in this case being between the mind, body, and soul. This union is achieved through the physical and spiritual practices of yoga, which include yoga postures, meditation, and pranayama (yogic breathing exercises). When practising yoga with complete devotion, this connection between the body and mind can ultimately lead to *samadhi*, or bliss.

## Yoga Philosophy – The Eight Limbs of Yoga

The practice of yoga does not just focus on physical postures to improve the body, but deals with all the aspects of our being. The 'eight limbs of yoga' are steps in a person's journey towards harmony of the mind, body, and spirit.

They are:

1. **YAMA:** our morals and ethical standards, and our behaviour towards others.

2. **NIYAMA:** our treatment of, and our attitude towards, ourselves.

3. **ASANA:** the regular practice of hatha yoga postures, through which we cultivate a healthy body and clear mind.

4. **PRANAYAMA:** a series of breath-control techniques that can lead to more efficient respiration, and highlight the connection between the breath, body, and mind.

5. **PRATYAHARA:** the practice of withdrawing the senses from the external world in order to turn focus inwards, increasing the focus on the mind.

6. **DHARANA:** the art of concentration which, when practised regularly, allows us to focus completely, remaining uninterrupted by external or internal distractions.

7. **DHYANA:** dharana (above) leads to dhyana, or meditation, a natural flow of energy between the self and the universe.

8. **SAMADHI:** the quiet state of blissful awareness, it is the culmination of the eight-limbed path of yoga.

⊚ Pigeon Pose, p.150

# The Chakras System

By working through the eight limbs of yoga we can balance our 'subtle body'. The subtle body is something you can't see or touch – it's where your energy flows. Chakras are believed to be the energy centres in the subtle body, lying within the spinal cord and corresponding to the main nerve centres in the body. As such, they affect both the subtle and physical body, transforming subtle energy into physical energy and back again.

There are seven main chakras and it is believed that by balancing our chakra system, we can lead healthier and happier lives.

The seven chakras are:

1. **MULADHARA:** the root chakra; located at the base of the spine.

2. **SVADHISTHANA:** the sacral chakra; located at the ovaries or prostate.

3. **MANIPURA:** the solar plexus chakra; located in the navel area.

4. **ANAHATA:** the heart chakra; located in the heart area.

5. **VISSUDHA:** the throat chakra; located in the throat and neck area.

6. **AJNA:** the brow or third eye chakra; located at the pineal gland (in the brain).

7. **SAHASRARA:** the crown chakra; located at the crown of the head.

Each chakra is located along the spine, starting at the base and running upwards, to the crown of the head. Each radiates a specific colour and spiritual quality, and together they make up the psychological, physical, and emotional states necessary for the development of the whole person. The three chakras residing below the heart are mainly concerned with the physical body and physical needs; the chakras above the heart are of a more spiritual nature.

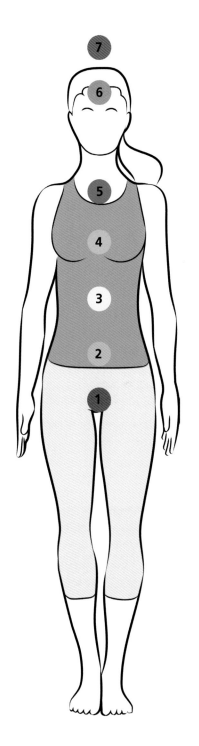

⊗ The seven chakras, and their position on the body.

# Origins and History of Yoga

Until recently, many Western scholars thought that yoga originated around 500 BCE, during the time of Gautama the Buddha. However, the discovery of engravings in the ruins of two cities of the Indus civilisation revealed that the origins reached back much further, to at least 5,000 years ago. Yoga has developed continuously since its origins and can be divided into five major periods: vedic yoga, pre-classical yoga, classical yoga, post-classical yoga, and modern yoga.

## Vedic Yoga

This Sanskrit word *veda* means knowledge. *The Vedas*, the scriptures from this period, comprise a collection of texts, songs, mantras, and rituals meant for use by a Vedic priest. The ancient yoga text the Rig Veda contains teachings about the praise of higher power and forms the origins of today's Hindu religion.

## Pre-classical Yoga

This covers the period from about 2000 BCE to the second century CE, during which the *Upanishads* were created. These philosophical texts teach about the sacrifice of the ego through self-knowledge, action, and wisdom, and the hidden unity of all things. They also contain the first reference to yoga as a path through which the student can gain freedom from suffering, and offer some instruction as to how this can be achieved.

## Classical Yoga

This relates to the period defined by Sage Patañjali's eight-limbed yoga, as taught in his text *The Yoga Sutra*. *The Yoga Sutra* was the first systematic presentation of yoga and has been scrutinised, interpreted, and commented on throughout the centuries since it was written. Patañjali presented the 'eight-limbed path', which outlines the stages towards obtaining enlightenment. The text is thought to have been written during the second century CE, and strongly influences many modern styles of yoga.

## Post-classical Yoga

Post-classical yoga differs from the yoga of other eras in that its goal is no longer liberation of the practitioner from their reality, but rather that they accept their own reality and attempt to live in the moment. Its teachings refer to *vedanta*, which represents a philosophical approach to the teachings of the Vedas, in particular, the Upanishads.

The yoga masters of this time created practices designed to rejuvenate and energise the body and prolong physical life. The ultimate aim of some of these practices was to energise the physical body to such a degree that the physical structure changed and the body became immortal. This is the origin of the modern yoga era, and of hatha yoga.

⊚ Warrior I Pose, p.70
The practice of asanas such as Warrior I became popular in the West during the twentieth century.

## Modern Yoga

This refers to the period in the nineteenth century during which numerous yoga masters brought their teachings to Europe and the United States. It was with the arrival of Swami Vivekananda, an Indian Hindu monk, in the United States, and his representation of India at the Parliament of World Religions in 1893, that the physical approach to yoga, known as hatha yoga, began to attract interest in the West.

Nearly thirty years later, in 1920, Paramahansa Yogananda arrived in Boston and established the Self-Realization Fellowship, which continues to have a wide following today. Other great modern teachers include Sri Krishnamacharya, who died at the age of 101 in 1989. His students included his son T.K.V. Desikachar, B.K.S Iyengar, Indra Devi, and Sri K. Pattabhi Jois. All these students became teachers and were very influential in spreading their knowledge of hatha yoga during the twentieth century. Their teachings are still practised throughout the world today.

## Hatha Yoga

Hatha yoga is the practice of asanas (yoga postures). The word 'hatha' comprises *ha* (meaning 'sun') and *tha* (meaning 'moon'), which refers to the balance of different aspects that are within all of us. This balance is achieved by regularly practising sequences of asanas which, as well as making the body strong and flexible, are intended to align the many energy channels of the body. In this way, hatha yoga is a path towards creating balance at all levels.

Many styles of hatha yoga are practised today – two of these, ashtanga yoga and Iyengar yoga, are especially popular in the West. These styles were popularised by Sri K. Pattabhi Jois and B.K.S. Iyengar respectively, and it is these two styles that form the basis of this book.

# Yoga and Breathing

Breathing is one physical function that, although involuntary – occurring as it does without instruction from our consciousness – can nevertheless be controlled. When we are not thinking about our breath, it continues to perform its vital functions of inhaling oxygen and exhaling carbon dioxide.

The nervous system is responsible for the regulation of breathing and controls the contractions of the muscles that make it happen. The process of breathing starts from a cluster of cells in the brain stem, collectively known as the respiratory centre, that send impulses to the muscles involved – the key muscles being the intercostals (between the ribs), and the diaphragm.

## Pranayama

Pranayama is a yogic practice that increases our awareness of the physical processes involved in breathing, and in doing so allows us to have more control over them.

With regular practice of breath control we can increase the amount of air we can take into the lungs, leading to increased oxygenation of the blood. This is thought to help repair the body at a cellular level. Controlling the breath through pranayama is known to lower both the heart rate and blood pressure, improving the efficiency of the body in utilising oxygen. When the body works efficiently in this way, it has less physical stress placed upon it. This allows the mind to become calm, and so easier to control – which is one of the main aims of yoga.

During the practice of yoga asana, we should aim to lengthen both the inwards breath and the outwards breath, subtly energising the body. Our breathing during yoga can also give an indication of whether we are working too hard and putting undue strain on the body. If the breath is shallow and erratic, the body is being overexerted and will become tense. This is a sign that the yoga practice should be gentler, so that the breath can again become slow and steady.

Lungs at rest

Inspiration

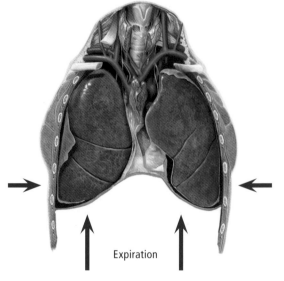

Expiration

# Breath-control Techniques

There are several pranayama techniques that can be used as part of a yoga practice. The two most common and accessible of these are outlined below:

### Victorious Breath (*Ujjayi* Breathing)

This technique is both energising and relaxing, and the sound it produces is often likened to the sound of the ocean. The breath is practised by inhaling slightly more deeply than normal and, with the mouth closed, exhaling through the nose. The muscles of the throat remain slightly constricted throughout, and this action of the throat creates a 'haaaa' sound. Ujjayi breathing can be performed in a seated position and is especially effective when done during asana practice.

### Alternate Nostril Breathing (*Nadi Shodhan*)

This is a simple breathing technique that works therapeutically to improve respiration and circulation. It also releases accumulated stress in the mind and body effectively.

Practise the breath by sitting comfortably with the spine straight and the left hand placed on the left knee, with the palm facing up. Tuck the tips of the index finger and middle finger of the right hand in towards the palm – if this is not possible, extend the fingers with the tips resting lightly on the 'third eye' point, in between the eyebrows. Close the right nostril with the thumb, and inhale through the left nostril. Then close the left nostril with the second finger and little finger, remove the thumb, and exhale through the right nostril. Inhale through the right nostril. Now press the thumb on the right nostril again, lift the second and little finger from the left nostril, and release the breath gently through the left nostril. This is one cycle of alternate nostril breathing.

This technique is usually practised for two minutes to begin with, gradually increasing to five minutes.

⊗ **Breathing**

When we breathe in, the intercostal muscles move the ribs upwards and outwards and the diaphragm pushes downwards. This draws air into the expanded lungs.

ⓥ During Shoulder Stand Pose (p.172) the 'chin-lock' position of the neck, and the effect of gravity pushing down on the diaphragm, encourage deep abdominal breathing.

# Yoga and the Spine

When viewed from the side, an adult spine has a natural S-shaped curve. The neck and lower back regions have a slight concave curve, and the thoracic and sacral regions have a slight convex curve. The purpose of these curves is to absorb shock, maintain balance, and allow range of motion throughout the spinal column.

For the spine to remain healthy, it is important that these natural curves of the spine are maintained. This can be achieved through the regular practice of a yoga programme that stretches and strengthens the spinal column as an entire unit.

Yoga creates flexibility around the vertebrae and intervertebral discs and strengthens the supportive network of muscles, ligaments, and tendons. Space is created between the vertebrae, easing pressure on the discs, while circulation is improved, helping regeneration at a cellular level. Bone density is also increased, helping to minimise degeneration of the bones.

A balanced yoga programme should include asanas that move the spine into and out of rotation, lateral flexion, forwards flexion, and extension. When all these types of movement are practised regularly, the spine will adopt a neutral alignment and negative postural patterns can be avoided. Good posture allows us to breathe more freely and improves our well-being by helping us to avoid muscle tightness and weakness that can contribute to backache.

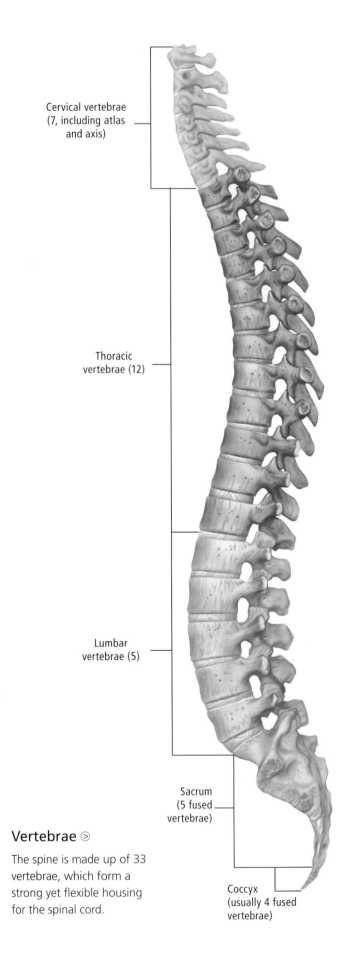

Cervical vertebrae
(7, including atlas
and axis)

Thoracic
vertebrae (12)

Lumbar
vertebrae (5)

Sacrum
(5 fused
vertebrae)

Coccyx
(usually 4 fused
vertebrae)

## Vertebrae ⊘

The spine is made up of 33 vertebrae, which form a strong yet flexible housing for the spinal cord.

# Joints and Movement

A well-balanced yoga programme should incorporate as many different ranges of movement as possible, so as to keep each joint functioning well. Within the skeleton there are three types of joints, which are categorised according to the degree of movement that each allows.

## Types of Joints

The bones of **fibrous joints** are connected by fibrous tissue that allows no movement (examples include where the bones of the skull join). The bones of **cartilaginous joints** are joined by cartilage. These joints must provide stability and so do not allow a great deal of movement. Examples include the sacroiliac joint, where the spine meets the pelvis, and the sternocostal joints, where the front ribs attach to the sternum (breast bone).

The bones of **synovial joints** meet in a joint capsule. Examples include the knee joint, where the femur and tibia meet, and the elbow joint, where the humerus meets with the radius and ulna. These joints are the most common and most mobile joints, and it is these that we will mostly be referring to in this book. The body has six types of synovial joints and their range of movement can be increased with regular hatha yoga practice.

ⓥ The three basic planes used to describe human anatomy.

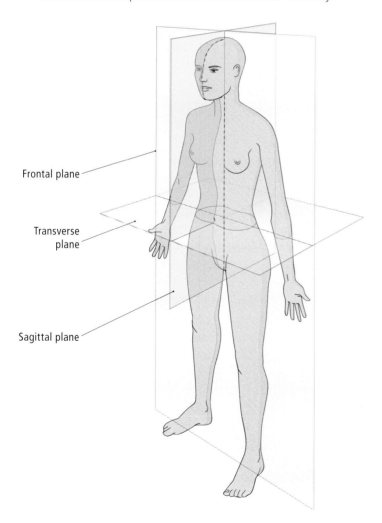

Frontal plane

Transverse plane

Sagittal plane

## Planes of Movement

Movements of the body can be categorised into types according to the direction in which they occur (see p.36). These types of movement also occur within a plane of movement. An anatomical plane is effectively an imaginary line – vertical or horizontal – drawn through the body.

There are three basic planes used in human anatomy:

**The frontal plane** is vertical and divides the body into back (posterior) and front (anterior) portions.

**The transverse plane** is parallel to the ground and separates the top half of the body from the lower half of the body.

**The sagittal plane** is vertical and divides the body into left and right portions.

These can be used to help describe movement – for example, by moving into Warrior I Pose (p.70), the front leg is in flexion at both the hip joint and knee joint, while the back leg is extended. Both of these movements occur in the sagittal plane. The arms are abducted out to either side and up overhead in a frontal plane. If the upper body then moved in to Revolved Side-angle Pose (p.82), the spine and torso would move on a transverse plane around a frontal axis point.

# Types of Muscle Activity

The muscles of the body are divided into three main types: skeletal, smooth, and cardiac. Skeletal muscles are those attached to the skeleton, and it is these that produce movement by shortening and pulling on a bone via its tendon – these are the muscles that we focus on in this book.

Most muscles work in opposing pairs to enable active extension and flexion in the joints – when one contracts and shortens, the other lengthens in response, and vice versa. When we stretch in hatha yoga, we are focusing mainly on muscles that lengthen as a result of another muscle shortening. For the purposes of hatha yoga, muscle contractions can be divided into two main types: isotonic and isometric.

## Isotonic Muscle Contraction

When a muscle changes length to create movement, it is called an isotonic contraction. Isotonic muscle contractions can be divided into either concentric or eccentric activity.

**Concentric** activity is when the muscle shortens to create movement. An example of this is bending the knee joint from straight to flexed, as in Shoulder Bridge Pose (p.168),

ⓥ Shoulder Bridge Pose, p.168
To achieve this bend at the knees, the hamstrings concentrically contract, acting as prime movers. The quadriceps must lengthen to allow this movement, acting as antagonists.

which causes a concentric contraction of the hamstring muscles. When a muscle creates a concentric contraction it is known as a **prime mover**, or **agonist**.

**Eccentric** muscle activity is when the muscle lengthens to allow movement. In the example above, to allow the knee to bend, the opposing muscles – the quadriceps – need to lengthen via an eccentric muscle contraction. An eccentric muscle is also known as an **antagonist**.

To create stable, co-ordinated movement, other muscles often contract or provide assistance to the prime mover. These muscles are known as **synergists**. For example, if the knee joint bends, the gastrocnemius muscle (located at the back of the lower leg) contracts to assist the hamstring muscles with this movement – in this case, the gastrocnemius works as a synergist.

## Isometric Muscle Contraction

Isometric contractions cause no change in the length of the muscle, but the muscle holds, or fixates, the body in position. For example, in Boat Pose (p.128), the rectus abdominis muscle group does not lengthen or shorten, but it contracts to hold the spine in place once the body has been moved into position. In this instance, the rectus abdominis muscle group would be known as a **fixator**.

⊗ Boat Pose, p.128
Once in this position, the rectus abdominis muscles (at the front of the abdomen) contract strongly to hold the body still, acting as fixators.

**In summary:**

- **Prime movers** produce the initial movement of a joint. These are also known as **agonists** and produce movement via a concentric contraction.

- **Antagonists** lengthen to allow the shortening of the prime mover, or agonist. This is an eccentric contraction.

- **Concentric muscle activity** – the muscle shortens to create movement (**prime movers**).

- **Eccentric muscle activity** – the muscle lengthens to allow movement (**antagonists**).

- **Synergists** contract to assist the prime mover.

- **Fixators** contract statically to stabilise the position adopted, once the movement has occurred.

For the purposes of the muscle activity examined in this book, the main muscle activity has been divided into **prime movers** – those that initiate the movement by shortening; and **antagonists** – those that allow the movement by lengthening.

# Levers and Intensity

The lever system is well established in physics, and it is an important factor in yoga – without levers movement could not occur, and they determine the intensity of each movement.

## What Is a Lever?

All levers are made up of three elements:

- an axis point, also known as a fulcrum
- a load, also known as resistance or weight
- an effort, also known as the force.

Collectively, the bones, ligaments, tendons, and muscles of the human body form levers to create movement. A joint forms the axis point and the muscles crossing the joint apply the effort, which then moves the lever, which in turn moves the load.

If we change the load or move the axis point, we change the effort the muscle has to exert to move the load. This means we can change the level of intensity levers experience, and so make particular movements of the body harder to achieve and maintain. An example of this outside of human anatomy is a children's see-saw. This has its axis point in the middle of the board and, because of this, the board will have an even load placed upon it (gravity) at either end. This means the board will remain parallel to the ground. If, however, we move the axis point to the left, for example, making the right side of the board longer, we have increased the load (gravity) at this end. The right side of the board will sink lower to the ground. This is a simple example of how moving the positioning of the axis changes the action of the lever.

## Types of Levers

There are three different types of lever in the human body: first-class levers, second-class levers, and third-class levers.

### First-class lever

A first-class lever has its axis located between the load and the effort. There are not many first-class levers in the human body, but one example is the joint between the head and the first vertebra of the neck. The load is the head, the axis is the joint, and the muscular action (effort) comes from the posterior muscles attaching to the skull, such as the trapezius. Therefore, if the upper trapezius muscles contract and shorten, they will be working against the weight of the head and gravity, and the chin will lift away from the chest and tilt backwards. An example of this can be found in Upward-facing Dog (p.146), where the chin is lifted a little.

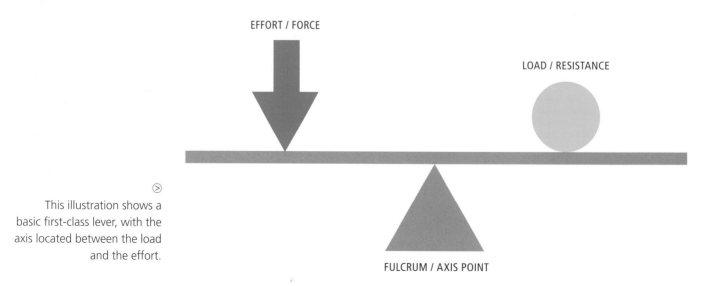

EFFORT / FORCE

LOAD / RESISTANCE

FULCRUM / AXIS POINT

⊘ This illustration shows a basic first-class lever, with the axis located between the load and the effort.

**Effort**

**Axis**

**Load**

⊙ Warrior II Pose, p.74
In this position, the arms each act as a third-class lever. The axis is the shoulder joint, the effort is applied by the deltoid muscles, and the load is the weight of the extended arm.

## Second-class lever

In a second-class lever, the load is located between the axis and the effort. A full press-up and the plank position are examples of this. The ankles are the axis point, the load is gravity, which is at its strongest at the centre of the body, and the effort is exerted predominantly from the deltoids, the muscles of the shoulders.

## Third-class lever

In a third-class lever, effort is applied between the load and the axis. By extending the arms out to either side, as in Warrior II Pose (p.74), the axis point is the shoulder joint. As we are not physically holding a weighted object, the load is created by gravity and the weight of the arm. The deltoids then exert the effort to keep the arms raised.

Another example of this is Warrior III Pose (p.104). The spine is in a forwards flexion position and the axis point is the sacroiliac joint at the base of the spine. As the arms are fully extended, the levers are long. This means that the load (gravity) placed upon the body is greater than if the hands were in front of the chest in Prayer Position, for example. The muscles that support the spine between the axis point (sacroiliac joint) and the hands then exert the effort – contract – to maintain the position of the spine.

# Modifications and Props

Yoga is a fundamentally accessible activity and can be practised in a variety of settings and places – it does not require much in the way of specialist equipment. However, there are a number of basic props you can use to help you get the most from your yoga practice. These can also help to make some asanas more attainable for those with limited mobility. Throughout the book we have provided suggestions for possible modifications to the asanas, with or without props.

## Yoga mat
A non-slip yoga mat is especially useful for standing poses where the feet are wide apart and there is a risk of slipping. They also act as padding in seated or lying poses. Using a mat can also improve your sense of spatial awareness.

## Yoga block
These are often used in seated poses to elevate the hips and move the lower back into a neutral alignment. For example, when in a Seated Forward Bend (p.124), if there is tightness in the lower back or hamstrings, the pelvis sometimes tilts back. By placing a yoga block underneath the hips, the hips can tilt forwards a little so the weight is directly on the sitting bones, straightening the spine.

## Yoga brick
A yoga brick is often used to place the hand on if it does not reach the floor. In Revolved Triangle Pose (p.66), for example, the left hand (when turning to the right) needs to be in contact with either the floor or a yoga brick to maintain stability. A yoga brick can also be used in a more supportive manner, such as being placed under the sacrum in Shoulder Bridge Pose (p.168) to support the lower spine, or under the top of the head when in a Wide-legged Forward Bend (p.114) to support the neck.

## Yoga belt
A yoga belt, depending on how it is used, can either assist in stretching muscles further or can support the body. To stretch the muscles more deeply in a Seated Forward Bend (p.124), for example, a yoga belt can be placed around the balls of the feet, increasing the resistance and so encouraging the ankle joint to stretch more intensely. The hamstring and calf muscles also stretch more in this instance. Adversely, a yoga belt placed around the lower back, inner thighs, and ankles while in Cobbler's Pose (p.136), will allow the legs and hips to relax while still being supported by the yoga belt.

⊘ Seated Forward Bend, p.124
This position can be modified with the help of a belt or strap placed around the balls of the feet, to create a more intense stretch.

## Blanket

A blanket can be used to provide padding for the body. For example, it can be placed underneath the hips in Boat Pose (p.128), or under the feet and ankles in Cobbler's Pose (p.136). It can also be used to cover the body in relaxation, simply to provide warmth.

## Wall

While not strictly a prop, a wall can be useful in learning poses that require a good deal of balance, such as Headstand Pose (p.180) or Half Moon Pose (p.100), as the wall can support the body and give the practitioner a sense of correct alignment. Some wide-legged forward bends can also be practised with the hands on a wall and the spine parallel to the floor, rather than placing the hands on the ground.

## Chair

Using a chair can be useful for those with limited mobility. For example, if moving to and from a seated position on the ground is not possible, a spinal twist could be performed sitting on the chair with the feet on the floor. The torso can then simply rotate to one side, with the left hand on the right knee and the right hand on the seat of the chair next to or behind the hips, before repeating on the other side.

ⓥ Yoga mats, bricks, and a yoga belt are shown below. Yoga bricks, often used to rest the hands on, are larger than yoga blocks, which can be placed beneath the hips during seated poses.

# Starting Poses

There are four starting poses used throughout this book, and these are explained below. You will be referred back to one of these at the beginning of most asanas.

## Mountain Pose
*Tadasana*

This is the foundation for all standing poses. Breathe steadily and stand upright with the arms by the sides and the feet together. Lift and spread the toes to help create a wide, solid base. Contract your thigh muscles so your kneecaps rise slightly, and draw the tail bone towards the floor to encourage neutral alignment of the pelvis and lumbar spine. Lift your sternum slightly, broadening the collarbone, and draw the shoulder blades downwards. Elongate the neck so that the crown of the head rises towards the sky and the chin is parallel to the ground.

## Staff Pose
*Dandasana*

Begin in a seated position with the legs extended in front of the torso. The spine should be perpendicular to the ground with the upper body extending upwards through the crown of the head. Place the palms of the hands on the ground on either side of the body, in-line with the hips, with the shoulders rolling back and down. Press the legs together and point the toes upwards with the feet in a neutral position. Contract the abdominal muscles lightly to support the spine and keep the chin level with the ground.

## Box Pose

Begin on the hands and knees, with the thighs at right-angles to the back, and the arms perpendicular to the ground. Ensure the knees are set directly below the front of the hips and there is a space in between the knees. Align the shoulders directly over the elbows and wrists, and spread out the fingers and thumbs. Position the entire spine, including the neck, parallel to the ground. The eyes should be looking at the floor, with the crown of the head pointing directly forwards.

## Corpse Pose
*Savasana*

This may look like a simple relaxing pose, done in between or after an asana, but it requires considerable concentration that develops through continued practice. Lie on the back with the legs straight and the feet hip-width apart. Allow the feet to fall gently out to either side, and rest the arms alongside the body, slightly separated from the body, with the palms facing upwards. Stretch through the body and draw the shoulder blades gently towards one another so the sternum lifts slightly. Start to breathe deeply, and watch the breath. If this asana is being used for final relaxation, stay here for several minutes.

# Standing Poses

Most yoga sequences involve standing poses and these often make up a considerable part of a balanced hatha yoga practice. This is largely due to their effectiveness in warming up the muscles of the body and the ligaments and tendons of the joints, helping to prepare for asanas that stretch them more deeply, while reducing the risk of injury. Longer-term benefits include increased overall strength, flexibility, and stability, particularly of the ankles, hips, and knees.

It is advisable that beginners in yoga focus mainly on standing yoga asanas to improve flexibility and posture of the spine, in order to create a good physical foundation before moving on to the more challenging asanas.

# Chair Pose

## Utkatasana

Chair Pose, also known as Fierce Pose, is a powerful asana that mimics sitting on a chair. It strengthens the whole body, particularly the back, legs, and all the major joints of the body. To achieve this position, the hip flexors contract and shorten while the quadriceps lengthen, creating a slight forwards tilt of the pelvis. The shoulder and upper back muscles work to raise the arms and draw the shoulder blades down. The larger muscle groups of the back then assist in maintaining the extension of the arms and the spine.

In this squat-like position, the shoulders, hips, knees, and ankles are all strengthened. For this reason, Chair Pose is useful to those who need to build up their strength before practising stronger standing asanas, and it can be useful to practise when recovering from knee and ankle injuries, as it builds stability in these joints. In addition, as Chair Pose utilises several muscles at the same time, the heart rate is increased, resulting in improved circulation and stamina.

## Level

Beginner

## Benefits

This asana strengthens all the major joints, including the shoulders, hips, knees, and ankles. It also improves stamina and muscle endurance.

## Caution

Practitioners with lower back injuries or high blood pressure should exercise caution when attempting this pose.

## ⊕ Modifications and props

To lower the intensity of the pose, reduce the bend of the knees, and instead of extending the arms upwards, place the hands in front of the chest in Prayer Position.

The feet can be positioned hip-width apart if balance is an issue, but care must be taken to keep the knees in line with the ankle joints.

##  Try to

Draw the pelvis downwards as the knees bend, maintaining a neutral position through the lumbar spine and an even weight through the feet.

Press the legs together to create a sense of strength through the lower body.

Draw the shoulders down, away from the head, to create space across the shoulders.

##  Try not to

Do not round the spine in any way, including overarching through the lumbar spine. Instead, draw the coccyx down towards the ground.

If the spine moves into a concave position when the arms are raised, take the arms slightly wider than shoulder-width apart. This will help to ensure neutral alignment of the spine.

# How to do it

### ⊘ **Step 1**

Begin in Mountain Pose (p.54).

### **Step 2** ⊘

Press the feet and legs together and exhale while bending the knees so that the legs adopt a squat position. Spread the toes and ensure the heels remain on the ground, with the weight evenly distributed through the feet. The chin should be parallel to the ground and the arms by the sides.

### ⊘ **Step 3**

On an inhale, sweep the arms upwards so they are in line with the ears and shoulder-width apart. The fingers and thumb of each hand should be closed together, not splayed. Now draw the shoulder blades down away from the head to create space across the top of the shoulders. Draw the coccyx downwards to help elongate the lumbar spine region, and contract the lower abdominal muscles to assist in supporting the lower back. Lift the sternum and chin a little to create a sense of lift through the upper body, and breathe steadily.

# Chair Pose

## Utkatasana

In Chair Pose there are many muscle groups working concentrically, eccentrically, and as fixators. The rectus femoris and the iliopsoas contract concentrically, helping to stabilise the pelvis. The erector spinae and quadratus lumborum lengthen eccentrically to allow the flexion of the spine, before fixating it in extension. The knees are partially flexed, shortening the hamstrings. The deltoids fixate the arms overhead while the triceps maintain the extended position of the elbows. The dorsiflexion of the feet occurs when the tibialis anterior and gastrocnemius shorten concentrically and the soleus muscles contract eccentrically. The abdominal muscles, in particular, the rectus and transversus abdominis, act as stabilisers of the torso.

**muscle activity**

**prime mover**

1   Rectus femoris
2   Iliopsoas
3   Adductor longus
4   Pectoralis major and minor
5   Anterior deltoids
6   Lower trapezius
7   Erector spinae
8   Triceps
9   Latissimus dorsi

**antagonist**

10   Rhomboids
11   Quadratus lumborum
12   Rectus abdominis
13   Vastus lateralis
14   Vastus intermedius
15   Vastus medialis
16   Gluteus maximus

(7 beneath thoracolumbar fascia;
14 beneath rectus femoris)

**spine**

The pelvis is in an anterior tilt position, with the spine moving into extension at the final phase of the asana. The spine extends forwards, moving in a sagittal plane from a medial lateral axis.

# Anatomy of the pose

Triceps 8

5 Anterior deltoids

4 Pectoralis major and minor

Latissimus dorsi 9

12 Rectus abdominis

Iliopsoas
(inside hip area, deep) 2

Gluteus maximus 16

14 Vastus intermedius

3 Adductor longus

1 Rectus femoris

Vastus lateralis 13

15 Vastus medialis

Not visible from this view:
(all on back)

6 Lower trapezius
7 Erector spinae
10 Rhomboids
11 Quadratus lumborum

# Triangle Pose

## Trikonasana

Triangle Pose is a basic yoga posture that is commonly practised in all styles of yoga. It stretches all the major joints, including the spine, shoulders, and hips. The spine is in a deep side-bend and the legs are apart, so the body creates several triangles, the lines of which are strong and straight. This results in an intense stretch of several major muscles groups. The inner thigh of the front leg and outer thigh of the back leg are stretched, as are the hamstrings of both legs. The weight of the upper body is mainly over the front leg, so the back leg, foot, and lower back muscles have to work hard to maintain the body's balance. With the spine positioned in a deep side-bend, the oblique abdominal muscles shorten on the right side of the torso and lengthen on the left side, increasing the overall strength of the core area. The arms are stretched away from the body and extend in opposite directions, with the right hand resting lightly on the ground behind the middle of the lower leg.

## Level

Beginner

## Benefits

This asana stretches and strengthens the legs; in particular, it works the muscles around the knees, ankles, hips, groin, and the hamstrings. It also opens the shoulders and chest.

Triangle Pose can help alleviate back pain by mobilising the spine and stretching the surrounding muscles.

## Caution

Due to the side-bend of the lumbar spine, those with lower back injuries and/or conditions should practise this asana with caution.

Triangle Pose should be modified for those with neck injuries or groin strain.

## ⊕ Modifications and props

For back injuries, bend the right knee slightly and/or rest the left hand behind the lower back, so the back of the hand is against the back of the lumbar region.

For neck injuries, keep the chin in line with the sternum (as opposed to looking upwards).

##  Try to

Press firmly through both feet to work both legs equally.

Contract the abdominal muscles to support the lumbar spine, especially when moving in and out of the posture.

Move the left shoulder and hip back slightly, so the left shoulder stacks on top of right and the chest area feels open.

##  Try not to

Do not allow the spine to pass lower than parallel to the upper body, as this will mean length in the upper body is lost. Instead, lengthen from the coccyx to the crown of the head.

Visualise a wall to the front and one behind. Stack the shoulders and hips so they do not touch the imaginary walls.

# How to do it

### ⌃ Step 1

Begin in Mountain Pose (p.54).

### ⌃ Step 2

Step the feet apart approximately 1.5 metres and extend the arms to either side so that they are parallel to the floor. Extend into the fingertips while drawing the shoulder down and check that the feet are aligned under the wrists. Turn the left toes in forty-five degrees and the right foot out ninety degrees. The heels should be in line with one another.

### ⌃ Step 3

Draw the spine upwards and, with the arms still parallel to the floor, move the spine into a side-bend, so that the mid- and upper torso are parallel to the ground. Ensure the arms are perpendicular to the ground, with the right hand resting lightly on the ground behind the middle of the tibia. Reach the left arm directly upwards.

### ⌃ Step 4

Now move the left shoulder and hip back slightly and tuck the right hip under a little. This will create more of a stretch along the left side of the torso. Rotate the neck in order to rest the gaze towards the left hand.

# Triangle Pose

## Trikonasana

To allow for the deep sideways bend of the spine in Triangle Pose, the iliopsoas, gluteus minimus, piriformis, and quadratus femoris of the right leg have to externally rotate the femur to create the space in the right hip joint for the right ilium bone to laterally tilt. It is this action that allows the hamstrings to lengthen, the gluteus maximus and hip flexors and quadriceps to extend the legs, and the adductors and abductors to lengthen. The lengthening through the right side is increased via an eccentric contraction of the gluteus medius and peroneus longus when the outer left foot presses firmly into the ground. The obliques lengthen eccentrically on the left side while concentrically contracting on the right side, and the mid-deltoids abduct the arms away from the medial line, while the triceps extend the elbows. The scapulae are retracted towards the spine, while the lower trapezius draws them away from the head. The sternocleidomastoid externally rotates the neck.

**muscle activity**

**prime mover**

1  External and internal obliques
2  Quadratus lumborum
3  Gluteus minimus
4  Piriformis
5  Quadratus femoris
6  Quadriceps
7  Triceps
8  Deltoids (mid-section)
9  Sternocleidomastoid

**antagonist**

10  Rectus abdominis
11  Iliopsoas
12  Peroneus longus
13  Trapezius

(2 beneath thoracolumbar fascia;
4 and 5 beneath gluteus maximus)

**spine**

The spine is in right lateral flexion, moving in a frontal plane from a sagittal axis. The pelvis is in a lateral tilt to the right.

# Anatomy of the pose

Not visible from this view:
(all on back)

2 Quadratus lumborum
3 Gluteus minimus
4 Piriformis
5 Quadratus femoris
13 Trapezius

Triceps
(other side of arm) 7

Deltoids (mid section) 8

1 External and internal
obliques

10 Rectus abdominis

6 Quadriceps

11 Iliopsoas
(deep)

Sternocleidomastoid 9

12 Peroneus longus

# Revolved Triangle Pose

## Parivrtta Trikonasana

This is a complex asana that improves flexibility and stability of all the major joints, particularly the hips, and the ability of the torso muscles to rotate the spine. It is very effective for improving posture, energy levels, and function of the internal organs, particularly the digestive system. It is also very effective in improving balance and awareness of space. The lower body is required to act as a strong foundation; the quadriceps are worked and the hamstrings stretched, so the spine can flex forwards. The spine can then twist freely while the major muscle groups of the back, including the latissimus dorsi and the oblique abdominal muscle groups, stretch and provide stability simultaneously.

When the spine moves into Revolved Triangle Pose, it is in a rotated forward-bend position. While this is generally beneficial, the spine can become vulnerable to injury if the practitioner pushes past their natural range of movement. Care should be taken to allow the muscles to stretch and release slowly.

### Level

Intermediate

### Benefits

This asana stretches and strengthens the hips, hamstrings, and calf muscles, and it opens the shoulders and chest to facilitate better breathing. Lower back pain is reduced and balance and stability of the entire body is improved.

### Caution

Practitioners with lower back injuries and/or back conditions should practise this asana with caution. Revolved Triangle Pose should be modified for those with neck injuries, groin strain, or low blood pressure.

### ⊕ Modifications and props

If the hand does not comfortably reach the floor, place a yoga brick underneath it. This will help maintain even length through either side of the torso, helping to stretch the spine.

If the torso does not rotate fully to the right, keep the chin in line with the sternum to avoid neck injury. The feet can also be positioned in a slightly diagonal stance, if it is difficult to align the pelvis correctly.

###  Try to

Lower the spine, so it is parallel to the ground, and stretch all the way to the crown of the head. This will create space along the spine and enable better breathing.

Press the outer edge of the left foot down and firmly contract the quadriceps muscles of both legs to increase the sense of balance and stability in the lower body.

Rotate the upper body slowly, moving the right hip back a little at the same time, to create space in the hips.

###  Try not to

Avoid resting heavily on the left hand. The left hand should rest lightly on the ground, ensuring the muscles around the waist work to support the lumbar region.

Try not to let the right shoulder drop forwards; instead, draw the right shoulder back so it is directly in line with the left shoulder. This will open the chest and neck area.

# How to do it

### ⊙ Step 1

Begin in Mountain Pose (p.54).

### ⊙ Step 2

On an exhale, step the feet approximately 1 metre apart and place the hands on the hip bones. Turn the left foot forty-five degrees to the right and the right foot ninety degrees to the right. Ensure the heels are aligned. Breathe steadily while you turn the torso and hips to the right, so the right and left front hip bones are in line with each other.

### ⊙ Step 3

Place the right hand on the lower back and extend the left arm directly upwards. Press firmly into the feet and contract the thigh muscles. Inhale, extending the spine upwards, then exhale while reaching the spine and left arm forwards until they are parallel to the ground.

### ⊼ Step 4

Inhaling, reach the left hand to the floor on the outside of the right foot. Keep pressing firmly into the edge of the back foot. Now begin to exhale and rotate the torso from the navel, so that the right shoulder stacks on top of the left shoulder. The neck should be parallel to the ground.

### ⊼ Step 5

Keep breathing deeply and move the right side of the hip bone back a little and extend the right arm upwards, with the palm of the hand facing outwards. The right and left arms should be in line with one another. Keep the neck long and rest the gaze on the right hand.

# Revolved Triangle Pose

## Parivrtta Trikonasana

To allow for the initial forwards flexion of the spine in Revolved Triangle Pose, the pelvis has to tilt forwards. This is achieved by the hip flexors, which shorten concentrically with the iliopsoas stabilising the pelvis. The hamstrings on the right and calf muscles (gastrocnemius and soleus) on the left lengthen eccentrically. The quadratus lumborum supports the lumbar region as it moves forwards, and the spine rotates due to the activation of the internal and external oblique muscles. The back foot presses firmly into the ground as the peroneus longus lengthens, helping the right side of the pelvis to align with the left side of the pelvis, bringing it level to the ground. The deltoids work to abduct the arms, while the triceps extend the arms from the elbow. The lower trapezius muscles draw the scapulae down and away from the head, which allows the head to turn more freely. The sternocleidomastoid externally rotates the neck.

**muscle activity**

**prime mover**

1  External and internal obliques
2  Sternocleidomastoid
3  Biceps femoris
4  Gluteus maximus and minimus
5  Triceps
6  Deltoids
7  Iliopsoas

**antagonist**

8   Adductors
9   Trapezius
10  Peroneus longus
11  Quadratus lumborum
12  Longissimus thoracis

(11 and 12 beneath thoracolumbar fascia)

**spine**

The spine is in forwards flexion and is rotated. It moves initially in a sagittal plane from a frontal axis, before rotating in a transverse plane. The pelvis is in an anterior tilt position.

# Anatomy of the pose

Triceps 5

Deltoids 6

9 Trapezius

12 Longissimus thoracis (beneath thoracolumbar fascia)

1 External and internal obliques

11 Quadratus lumborum (beneath thoracolumbar fascia)

4 Gluteus maximus and minimus

7 Iliopsoas (inside hip area, deep)

3 Biceps femoris

Sternocleidomastoid 2

8 Adductors

Peroneus longus 10

# Warrior I Pose

## Virabhadrasana I

Warrior I is an invigorating asana that is effective at increasing the range of movement of all the major joints. It encourages all the main muscle groups to work in synergy, which helps to open the hips and shoulders; strengthen the legs, arms, and back; and increase energy levels and mental focus.

The spine is in a slight backbending position, so it strengthens the extensors of the spine – mainly the erector spinae – and stretches the front of the upper body. The left leg is straight, so the hip flexors lengthen, while the right leg is bent and works powerfully with the quadriceps and adductors, which hold its position. This action of the legs helps to stretch and strengthen both sides of the hips and creates a strong foundation. The chest and front of the shoulders are open, so the arms can reach directly upwards. This creates a stretch and sense of lift through the entire upper body. Warrior I Pose can be practised within Sun Salutation sequences or as part of a standing sequence.

## Level

Intermediate

## Benefits

Warrior I is an energising asana that increases the heart rate and thus improves stamina. It stretches and strengthens the hip flexors, opens the chest and shoulders, and works the muscles of the back.

## Caution

Practitioners with lower back injuries and/or back conditions should practise this asana with caution. Warrior 1 Pose should be modified for those with neck injuries, groin strain, or low blood pressure.

### ⊕ Modifications and props

If the hips are inflexible, move the right foot to the right by 5–10 centimetres, to allow the pelvis and lower back to move more freely.

Separate the hands to shoulder-width apart if it is difficult to straighten the arms with the hands together.

For knee injuries, decrease the bend in the right leg; for neck injuries, look forwards.

###  Try to

Press the edge of the left foot down firmly into the ground and align the right knee directly over the ankle; this will help prevent overstretching of the knee tendons.

Draw the scapulae downwards to free up the neck.

Move the right front hip bone backwards, and the left one forwards.

###  Try not to

Never allow the right knee to move further forwards than directly over the ankle, or allow the right thigh to move inwards, so the knee is no longer over the ankle.

Do not force the left front hip bone forwards. The shoulders should not move upwards. Do not overextend the lumbar spine.

# How to do it

### ⌃ Step 1

Begin in Mountain Pose (p.54).

### ⌃ Step 2

On an inhale, take a big step backwards (approximately 1.5 metres) with the left foot. Turn the left foot out forty-five degrees, pressing the edge of the foot firmly into the ground. Exhale and bend the right knee to a right angle, so that the knee is aligned directly over the ankle. The ankles should be in line with each other.

### ⌃ Step 3

Breathing steadily, press firmly into the feet and align the front of the ribcage and pelvis to face forwards by moving the right hip back a little and the left hip gently forwards. Extend the spine upwards and gently contract the lower abdominal muscles to assist in supporting the lower back.

### ⌃ Step 4

Inhale and extend the arms directly upwards, so they are in line with the ears, and press the palms of the hands firmly together. Move the shoulders downwards, away from the head. Lift the gaze up to the hands by moving the chin away from the chest, being careful not to overarch the lower back. Keep breathing steadily throughout.

# Warrior I Pose

## Virabhadrasana I

During Warrior I Pose the right leg works powerfully, with the hip flexors and the hamstrings concentrically contracting. This moves the knee into a flexed position, with the quadriceps lengthening eccentrically, and the adductors and gluteal muscles fixating the leg. The left leg is extended back due to a concentric contraction of the quadriceps and left gluteus maximus, while the sartorius and biceps femoris create an external rotation of the femur. The peroneus longus and soleus activate the edge of the left foot to supinate it slightly. This action helps to concentrically contract the quadriceps and stretch the front of the left hip.

The spine extends upwards with the erector spinae shortening via a concentric contraction. The rectus abdominis and latissimus dorsi work to fixate this position. The deltoids initially extend the arms before fixating them in place, while the triceps extend the arms from the elbow. The trapezius draws the scapulae away from the head, allowing the neck to extend more freely.

**muscle activity**

**prime mover**

1  Hamstrings
2  Quadriceps
3  Sartorius
4  Gluteus maximus and minimus
5  Trapezius
6  Erector spinae
7  Triceps
8  Deltoids
9  Hip adductors

**antagonist**

10  Iliopsoas
11  Latissimus dorsi
12  Rectus abdominis
13  Peroneus longus
14  Soleus

(6 beneath thoracolumbar fascia)

**spine**

The spine is in extension with slight external rotation of the left hip and left lumbar region. This asana moves in a sagittal plane, with a slight movement in the transverse plane due to the external rotation of the left side. The spine moves from a frontal axis. The pelvis is in a slight anterior tilt.

# Anatomy of the pose

Triceps 7

Deltoids 8

Latissimus dorsi 11

Rectus abdominis 12

Hip adductors 9

Quadriceps 2

Sartorius 3

14 Soleus

5 Trapezius

6 Erector spinae

10 Iliopsoas
(inside hip area, deep)

4 Gluteus maximus and minimus

1 Hamstrings

Peroneus longus 13

# Warrior II Pose

## Virabhadrasana II

Warrior II is a standing asana that enhances posture, strength, stability, and concentration, and can be an effective way to build a feeling of inner strength. It uses all the major muscle groups and opens the hips, chest, and shoulders, while strengthening the legs, arms, and back.

The right knee joint is bent, with the knee aligned over the ankle, and the left leg is straight; therefore, the quadriceps shorten on the left side and lengthen on the right side. This helps to open the front of the hips while the iliopsoas muscles help to stabilise the pelvis. The spine is extended upwards and the chest area is broad and open. The arms are extended out strongly to either side, with the palms facing down, and the shoulder blades are drawing downwards as the upper back muscles gently contract. The neck extensors help to turn the head so the gaze can rest on the right hand. With so many muscle groups working hard, the heart rate and circulation are increased, making this a very energising asana.

## Level

Beginner

## Benefits

Warrior II Pose strengthens and stretches the legs, hips and ankles, and opens the chest area. It improves stamina by increasing the heart rate and circulation. The shoulders are also stretched and strengthened, and mental focus is increased.

## Caution

Practitioners with high blood pressure should be cautious when practising this asana.

Groin strain and knee and ankle injuries can be exacerbated when the full asana is practised; therefore, appropriate modifications should be used.

###  Modifications and props

For knee injuries, decrease the bend of the right knee; for lower back injuries, shorten the stance; and for sciatica, position the back foot at a ninety-degree angle.

For high blood pressure, position the hands in front of the chest in Prayer Position, so circulation is slowed.

### ⊘ Try to

Ensure the right knee is directly over the right ankle and the edge of the left foot is pressed down firmly, as this will help to stretch the left hip.

Elongate the spine to minimise pressure in the lower back, and keep the arms level, as this will help to strengthen the shoulders.

### ⊗ Try not to

Avoid stepping the feet too far apart as this could overstretch the hips and affect balance. Conversely, if the stance is too short, the right knee can become overstretched, so do not allow the right knee to move past the ankle.

Do not allow the shoulders to move upwards, as this will cause tension in the neck.

# How to do it

◁ **Step 1**

Begin in Mountain Pose (p.54).

⌃ **Step 2**

On an exhale, move the feet approximately 1.5 metres apart; then, inhaling, extend the arms out to either side, so that they are parallel to the ground. Ensure that the heels are aligned with one another, and that the feet are aligned directly under the hands.

◁ **Step 3**

Turn the right foot out ninety degrees and the left foot in forty-five degrees and align the right heel with the arch of the left foot. Then exhale while bending the right knee, moving the leg into a right-angled position. Ensure the right knee is aligned directly over the right ankle. The left leg should remain straight and the thigh should be firm. Breathing evenly, press the outer left foot firmly into the floor and draw the coccyx downwards to lengthen the lower back. Draw the shoulder blades downwards and keep the arms strong. Rest the gaze towards the right hand, with the chin level to the floor.

# Warrior II Pose

## Virabhadrasana II

During Warrior II the spine is in extension, initiated by the erector spinae, with the latissimus dorsi and rectus abdominis working as fixators. The arms are abducted away from the medial line of the body and are parallel to the floor with the hands in pronation. While the triceps contract concentrically to extend the arms from the elbows, it is the deltoids that hold the arms in place. The hamstrings of the right leg shorten concentrically, creating flexion at the knee joint, and the quadriceps lengthen to allow this movement to occur. Conversely, the left leg is fully extended, with the gluteal muscles and quadriceps activated concentrically and the hip flexors lengthened eccentrically. The sartorius and biceps femoris of the left leg are the hip flexors that externally rotate the thigh and hip to create a stretch across the front of the pelvis and in the adductors. It is the peroneus longus that lengthens as the outer left foot presses firmly in to the ground. The scapulae are retracted towards the spine while the trapezius draws them away from the head. The sternocleidomastoid rotates the head and neck.

**muscle activity**

**prime mover**

1 Hamstrings
2 Quadriceps
3 Adductors
4 Gluteus maximus and medius
5 Sartorius
6 Erector spinae
7 Triceps
8 Deltoids
9 Trapezius

**antagonist**

10 Latissimus dorsi
11 Rectus abdominis
12 Iliopsoas
13 Peroneus longus

(6 beneath thoracolumbar fascia)

**spine**

The spine is in extension, moving in a frontal plane from a sagittal axis.
The pelvis is in a neutral position.

# Anatomy of the pose

Not visible from this view:

4 Gluteus maximus and medius (rear of leg)
6 Erector spinae (on back)
7 Triceps (rear of arm)
9 Trapezius (on back)
10 Latissimus dorsi (on back)

Deltoids 8

Rectus abdominis 11

Iliopsoas 12

Sartorius 5

Quadriceps 2

1 Hamstrings

3 Adductors

Peroneus longus 13

# Extended Side-angle Pose

## Utthita Parsvakonasana

Extended Side-angle Pose is a strong asana that works all the major muscle groups and requires considerable flexibility of the major joints, in particular the hips and shoulders. For this reason, it is considered a 'master posture'.

With the left leg fully extended and the right knee flexed to a right angle, the legs create a strong foundation. The core muscles of the upper body work to fix the body in place. By reaching the left arm over to create a straight line, the entire left side of the body is stretched, increasing the flexibility of the ribcage. The flexibility of the lower back and hips can be increased further by moving the outer left hip back a little. This creates a deeper stretch on the left side of the body; however, it can sometimes be too intense for beginners and should therefore be practised with caution.

## Level

Intermediate

## Benefits

This asana strengthens and stretches the legs, hips, shoulders, and ankles.

It increases stamina by elevating the heart rate and improves respiration by stretching the lungs. Increasing the flexibility of the connective tissue of the ribcage allows for greater expansion and deeper breathing.

## Caution

Practitioners with high blood pressure should be cautious when practising this asana.

Groin strain and knee and ankle injuries can also be exacerbated when the full asana is practised; therefore, appropriate modifications should be used.

###  Modifications and props

For knee injuries, decrease the bend of the right knee. For lower back injuries and high blood pressure, shorten the stance and place the right forearm on the right thigh. For sciatica, position the back foot at a ninety-degree angle.

### ⊘ Try to

Ensure the right knee is directly over the right ankle and the edge of the left foot is pressed down firmly, as this will help to stretch the left hip.

Elongate the spine to minimise pressure in the lower back, and keep the arms level, as this will help to strengthen the shoulders.

### ⊗ Try not to

Try not to rest on the right hand or forearm.

# How to do it

### ⊘ Step 1

Begin in Mountain Pose (p.54).

### ⊘ Step 2

On an exhale, move the feet approximately 1.5 metres apart. Next, extend the arms out to either side, so that they are parallel to the ground. Ensure that the heels align and the feet are aligned directly under the hands.

### Step 3 ⊘

Inhale while turning the right foot out ninety degrees and the left foot in forty-five degrees, and align the right heel with the arch of the left foot. Exhale and bend the right knee, moving the leg into a right-angled position. Ensure that the right knee is directly over the right ankle.

### ⊼ Step 4

Now extend the torso to the right, placing the right hand on the ground behind the right leg. Inhale and extend the left arm up to align with the left ear, creating a long straight line from the edge of the left foot to the left fingertips. Face the palm of the left hand towards the ground.

### ⊼ Step 5

Move the left hip back slightly as the right hip moves forwards, increasing the stretch in the hips. Maintain the strength through the legs and abdominal muscles, so that the right arm does not have to support the posture. Bring the gaze to the left hand and breathe steadily.

# Extended Side-angle Pose

## Utthita Parsvakonasana

To allow for the deep flexion of the right knee in Extended Side-angle Pose, the hamstrings shorten and the quadriceps lengthen, while the adductors assist to fix the leg in position. The left leg is fully extended and the concentric contraction of the quadriceps is maximised by the peroneus longus lengthening and helping to press the edge of the left foot in to the ground. The hip flexors, sartorius, and biceps femoris then externally rotate the left leg and hip slightly, helping to open the entire left side of the body. The hamstrings of the left leg now lengthen eccentrically.

The spine is in deep lateral flexion to the right, achieved by the obliques and quadratus lumborum on the right side of the body, as they contract concentrically. The latissimus dorsi and rectus abdominis then fixate the upper body in place. The arms are abducted away from the medial line by the deltoids, with the left arm extended over the head via a concentric contraction of the serratus anterior. The pectorals lengthen eccentrically. The scapulae are retracted towards the spine while the trapezius draws them away from the head. The sternocleidomastoid rotates the neck.

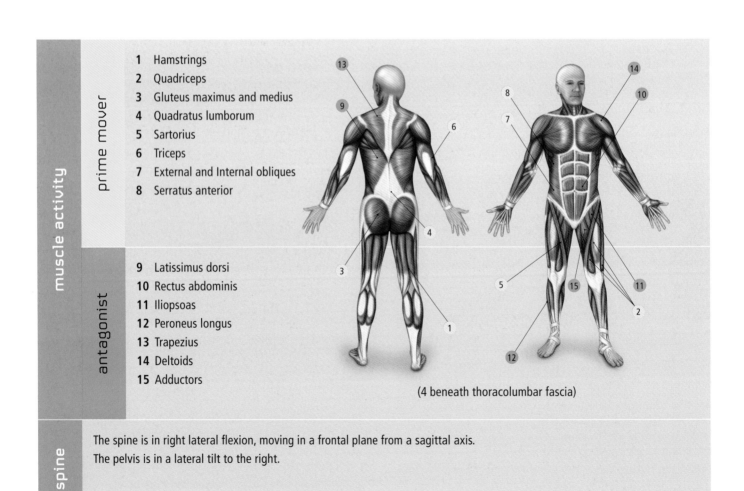

**muscle activity**

**prime mover**

| | |
|---|---|
| 1 | Hamstrings |
| 2 | Quadriceps |
| 3 | Gluteus maximus and medius |
| 4 | Quadratus lumborum |
| 5 | Sartorius |
| 6 | Triceps |
| 7 | External and Internal obliques |
| 8 | Serratus anterior |

**antagonist**

| | |
|---|---|
| 9 | Latissimus dorsi |
| 10 | Rectus abdominis |
| 11 | Iliopsoas |
| 12 | Peroneus longus |
| 13 | Trapezius |
| 14 | Deltoids |
| 15 | Adductors |

(4 beneath thoracolumbar fascia)

**spine**

The spine is in right lateral flexion, moving in a frontal plane from a sagittal axis.
The pelvis is in a lateral tilt to the right.

# Anatomy of the pose

**Not visible from this view:**

3 Gluteus maximus and medius (rear of leg)
4 Quadratus lumborum (on back)
9 Latissimus dorsi (on back)
13 Trapezius (upper back)

6 Triceps

14 Deltoids

8 Serratus anterior

10 Rectus abdominis

7 External and internal obliques

11 Iliopsoas

12 Peroneus longus

15 Adductors

2 Quadriceps

5 Sartorius

1 Hamstrings

# Revolved Side-angle Pose

## Parivrtta Parsvakonasana

Revolved Side-angle Pose is an asana that requires a great level of flexibility and strength. It is very effective in increasing the mobility of all the major joints and the entire spine, and it increases flexibility of the thoracic region in particular. The legs work hard and the front of the hips are stretched deeply, allowing the pelvis to move into the correct alignment. The left leg is fully extended and the right knee is flexed to a right angle, creating a strong foundation for the upper body. The core muscles work powerfully to rotate the upper body, and, as a result of this rotation, the internal organs, including the digestive system, are stimulated, creating a detoxifying effect.

The flexibility of the spine and hips can be increased further with a small external rotation of the right shoulder. This creates a deeper stretch on the right side of the body. However, this can be too intense for practitioners with injuries and should be practised with caution.

### Level

Advanced

### Benefits

This asana stretches the entire body and strengthens the legs, shoulders, and ankles. The hips, in particular, are stretched, while the heart rate is increased, improving respiration.

The rotation of the spine also momentarily compresses some of the internal organs, which stimulates digestion.

### Caution

Practitioners with injuries to the vertebral discs should not practise this asana.

Those with other lower back issues or knee injuries should modify this asana.

### ⊕ Modifications and props

To modify this asana, a brick can be placed under the left hand and the right hand can be placed on the lower back; this will decrease the range of motion.

To decrease the rotation of the spine, the left arm can be placed on the inside of the right leg.

###  Try to

Ensure the right arm is parallel to the ground and try to create as much length through the spine as possible before rotating the upper body.

Rest the left hand lightly on the ground and maintain strength through the legs and abdominal muscles.

Create a long straight line from the edge of the left foot to the right fingertips.

###  Try not to

Avoid resting heavily on the left hand, as this will build pressure in the wrist.

Avoid lifting the edge of the back foot from the floor and resting the upper body on the right thigh.

Do not strain the neck in order to look at the right hand. Instead, if uncomfortable, keep the chin in line with the sternum.

# How to do it

⊘ **Step 1**

Begin in Mountain Pose (p.54).
(Steps 1–3 viewed from the front)

⊼ **Step 2**

Step the feet approximately 1.5 metres apart; then, on the next inhale, reach the arms out to either side, so that they are parallel to the floor.

⊼ **Step 3**

Turn the right foot out forty-five degrees and the left foot in ninety degrees. Exhaling, bend the right leg to a right angle, aligning the knee over the ankle.

⊼ **Step 4**

(Steps 4–6 viewed from the side)
Rotate the upper body to the right and extend the spine over the right thigh at the same time. Keep pressing the left foot firmly down into the ground and sink the right hip back as the left hip moves forwards a little. Keep reaching the arms out to the sides.

⊼ **Step 5**

Place the right hand on the lower back and, on an exhale, rotate the upper body deeply to the right, placing the left arm to the outside of the right leg, in line with the lower leg and ankle. Once the left hand is on the ground, pause and inhale, and then, while exhaling, rotate further still, so that the right shoulder now aligns over the left shoulder.

⊼ **Step 6**

Breathing steadily, extend the right arm upwards, before exhaling as you extend it over the head, so that it is in line with the right ear. Really stretch from the edge of the left foot all the way to the fingertips on the right hand, to get a deep stretch in the right side of the ribcage. Rest the gaze towards the right hand.

# Revolved Side-angle Pose

## Parivrtta Parsvakonasana

In Revolved Side-angle Pose, the left knee is flexed, with the hamstrings and hip flexors shortening concentrically and the quadriceps lengthening eccentrically. These actions are reversed on the right leg, with the hamstrings lengthening eccentrically and quadriceps shortening, leading to full extension of the knee. The adductors work to stabilise both legs, while the iliopsoas supports the pelvis. There is also an inwards rotation of the right leg as the upper body rotates to the left. The entire spine, but particularly the thoracic spine, deeply rotates due to a strong concentric contraction of the latissimus dorsi and internal and external obliques. To support this position, the quadratus lumborum supports the lumbar region, while the rectus abdominis assists to fixate the upper body. The triceps extend the arms from the elbows, while the deltoids and serratus anterior work to extend the left arm over the head. The trapezius retracts the scapulae and the sternocleidomastoid externally rotates the neck.

**muscle activity**

**prime mover**

| | |
|---|---|
| 1 | External and Internal obliques |
| 2 | Latissimus dorsi |
| 3 | Sartorius |
| 4 | Biceps femoris |
| 5 | Gluteus maximus and minimus |
| 6 | Serratus anterior |
| 7 | Triceps |
| 8 | Deltoids |
| 9 | Hamstrings |

**antagonist**

| | |
|---|---|
| 10 | Iliopsoas |
| 11 | Adductors |
| 12 | Trapezius |
| 13 | Peroneus longus |
| 14 | Quadratus lumborum |

(14 beneath thoracolumbar fascia)

**spine**

The spine moves initially into a lateral flexion, moving in a frontal plane from a sagittal axis.
The spine then externally rotates to the right in a transverse plane from a sagittal axis.
The pelvis is in an anterior tilt.

# Anatomy of the pose

**Not visible from this view:**

2  Latissimus dorsi (on back)
11  Adductors (inner thigh)
12  Trapezius (upper back)

Serratus anterior  6

External and
internal obliques  1

Quadratus lumborum
(beneath  14
thoracolumbar fascia)

Gluteus maximus
and medius  5

Iliopsoas (inside  10
hip area, deep)

7  Triceps

3  Sartorius

4  Biceps femoris

9  Hamstrings

13  Peroneus longus

8  Deltoids

# Standing Balancing Poses

These asanas are often practised once the body is warm. They greatly improve the strength of the knees and ankles. This is largely due to the small stabilising muscles and connective tissues in and around the joints becoming active in stabilising the knee and ankle, so that the participant does not lose their balance. Furthermore, all asanas that involve an element of balance will greatly improve mental focus and clarity, as concentration is required to practise these poses effectively.

# Tree Pose

## Vrksasana

Tree Pose is a balancing asana that greatly improves the strength, flexibility, and stability of all the major joints. The left leg is straight, with the knee joint fully extended, and the quadriceps work hard to hold the leg in place. The adductors and gluteal muscles also assist with this action. The hip flexors lift the right thigh towards the upper body and move it outwards from the hip joint, so the right foot can rest on the left inner thigh. The hip flexors contract to help support the pelvis and lumbar region during these actions. The spine is elongated and, as there is no movement forwards, backwards, or to either side in this asana, it is in a neutral position. The arms reach overhead with the hands pressed firmly together, giving a sense of lift and lightness, and the sacral region is drawn downwards to counteract possible overextension of the lumbar region when the arms are extended. Maintaining this stance helps to slow down erratic or fast-paced breathing, lowers the heart rate and calms the nervous system. It creates a sense of stillness in mind and body.

## Level

Beginner

## Benefits

Tree Pose improves postural awareness and alignment.

It encourages the practitioner to focus on their breathing, which in turn improves mental focus and rejuvenates the mind and body.

## Caution

For those with high blood pressure or ankle or knee injuries, the asana should be modified and practised with cautions. Care should also be taken for those with sciatica.

 **Modifications and props**

For high blood pressure, place the hands in Prayer Position in front of the chest.

For ankle or knee injuries, place the raised foot on the inside of the ankle of the opposite leg, with the toes touching the floor, to offer more support.

Those who struggle to balance can practise Tree Pose using a wall for support.

⊘ **Try to**

Ensure both legs feel strong and keep the hips level with one another, so both sides of the lower back are working equally. Keep the chin level to the floor and draw the shoulders downwards.

Feel a sense of lightness through the body by reaching upwards and elongating the spine.

Ensure the right foot is placed on the left inner thigh; avoid placing the foot on the inside of the knee joint.

 **Try not to**

Try not to lift the shoulders towards the head when the arms are raised. If the shoulders are lifting, separate the hands instead and move the shoulder blades down.

Try not to bend the left knee and instead focus on straightening the knee and contracting the quadriceps.

# Anatomy of the pose

## ⌃ Step 1

Begin in Mountain Pose (p.54).

## ⌃ Step 2

Transfer the weight to the left foot and contract the muscles of the left thigh. Now, press down into the left foot, exhale, and place the right foot on the inside of the left inner thigh, placing the right hand around the right ankle to move the foot into position. The right knee should be bent and pointing out to the side, and the hips should be level with one another. Press the right foot firmly into the left inner thigh and relax the toes.

## ⌃ Step 3

Inhale while lifting the hands to chest height, pressing them together in Prayer Position. The elbows should be pointing down towards the ground and the shoulders should be relaxed. Pause here and breathe.

## ⌃ Step 4

Inhale again while extending the arms upwards, until the hands are directly over the head, still in Prayer Position. The elbows should be slightly bent and the shoulders drawn downwards. Straighten the spine upwards, relax the face and look forwards with the chin level to the floor.

# Tree Pose

## Vrksasana

Throughout Tree Pose, the spine is in a neutral position and is supported by the major muscles surrounding the thoracic and lumbar region. These include the erector spinae and abdominal muscles, which are contracted isometrically. The arms are extended overhead when the deltoids contract concentrically. The triceps also work concentrically, while the biceps femoris lengthen eccentrically to extend the arms from the elbows, and the trapezius muscles retract the scapulae away from the head. The quadriceps of the left leg contract concentrically to fully extend the knee, while the stabilisers around the knees and ankle work powerfully to fixate these joints in place. The gluteal and abductors also work hard to stabilise the leg. The right femur is externally rotated from the hip joint when the gluteus minimus and hip flexors, sartorius, and biceps femoris shorten concentrically and the hamstrings shorten to flex the right knee. The iliopsoas shortens concentrically on the right side and fixates on the left side.

**muscle activity**

**prime mover**

| 1 | Iliopsoas |
| 2 | Quadriceps |
| 3 | Sartorius |
| 4 | Biceps femoris |
| 5 | Gluteus minimus |
| 6 | Deltoids |
| 7 | Triceps |

**antagonist**

| 8 | Gluteus maximus |
| 9 | Trapezius |
| 10 | Serratus anterior |

(5 beneath gluteus maximus)

**spine**

The spine is in a neutral position. The pelvis is also in a neutral position.
Therefore, no movement occurs in a plane or around an axis.

# Anatomy of the pose

7 Triceps

10 Serratus anterior

Quadriceps 2

1 Iliopsoas (deep)

Biceps femoris 4

3 Sartorius

**Not visible from this view:**

5 Gluteus minimus (rear)
6 Deltoids (outer side of shoulder)
8 Gluteus maximus (rear)
9 Trapezius (on back)

# Eagle Pose

## Garudasana

Eagle Pose is an invigorating asana that improves balance and co-ordination. It stretches the upper back and shoulders and strengthens all the major joints of the body. Due to the balancing elements of this asana, the knees and ankles are greatly strengthened, as they work hard to stabilise themselves. The hips, knees, and elbows are all flexed, causing a momentary restriction of the blood flow through the joints, which then results in improved circulation when the pose is released.

When the hands move away from the face and the shoulder blades move away from one another, the upper back muscles are stretched. The extensors of the spine contract, so the upper body remains upright. The legs are pressed together, strengthening the adductors and quadriceps and stretching the outer thigh. This in turn helps to maintain good alignment of the knee cap, which benefits the knee joint. Eagle Pose also stretches the gluteal muscles, which helps to ease lower back pain, and it also stretches the muscles that surround the sciatic nerve, helping to ease some cases of sciatica.

### Level

Beginner

### Benefits

This pose strengthens the ankles, knees, and hips, and stretches the shoulders. It improves core stability and can ease pain in the lower back.

### Caution

Those with knee, ankle, and shoulder injuries should practise this asana with caution.

Practitioners with low blood pressure should practise this asana gently and be careful not to overexert themselves.

### ⊕ Modifications and props

For knee and/or ankle injuries, place a yoga brick under the toes of the right foot or place the toes on the floor, to offer support to the injured joint.

If the shoulders are stiff or injured, place the right arm under the left and rest the backs of the hands together, instead of the palms.

### ⊘ Try to

Draw the shoulders downwards and align the hands and wrists directly over the elbows.

Move the knees to the centre line of the body, so they are aligned over the ankles, and press the legs together to improve stability.

### ⊗ Try not to

Try not to tighten the shoulders by allowing the scapulae to lift.

Do not lean forwards; instead, extend the spine upwards.

Do not force the right foot behind the left calf muscle, as this may injure the knee; instead, rest the foot gently on the left lower leg.

# How to do it

### ⊘ Step 1

Begin in Mountain Pose (p.54).

### Step 2 ⊘

Inhale and stretch the arms straight out in front of the body, so they are parallel to the ground. While exhaling, sweep the right arm underneath the left arm, bending the elbows at the same time. Now inhale and press the palms of the hands together. The fingers and thumbs should be pointing upwards with the forearms perpendicular to the floor.

### Step 3 ⊘

Exhaling, move into a squat position by pressing the legs and feet together and bending the knees, keeping the heels firmly on the ground and extending the spine upwards. Press the thighs together and tilt the pelvis forwards slightly. Draw the abdominal muscles in towards the spine.

### ⊘ Step 4

Keeping the left leg bent, inhale while lifting the right leg up and over the left leg, placing the right thigh on top of the left thigh. Tuck the right foot behind the left lower leg so the right toes are pointing downwards. Draw the crown of the head is upwards, extending the spine. The gaze should be directly forwards, with the chin level to the floor. Breathe steadily.

# Eagle Pose

## Garudasana

In Eagle Pose, the hamstrings are concentrically contracted and the quadriceps lengthened eccentrically, causing flexion at the knee. The iliopsoas, sartorius, and biceps femoris all shorten, causing flexion at the hips. This in turn moves the spine into forwards flexion before the erector spinae shortens concentrically, creating a slight extension in the lumbar spine. The right ankle joint is plantarflexed, while the left ankle is dorsiflexed, and the adductors work hard to press the thighs together. This results in the femurs both rotating internally. The gluteal muscles work to stabilise the hips, and the abdominal muscles – mainly the rectus abdominis – assist to fixate the upper body in place. The pectorals and anterior deltoids draw the arms towards one another, while the trapezius and rhomboids draw the scapulae downwards, creating a stretch across the upper back and neck.

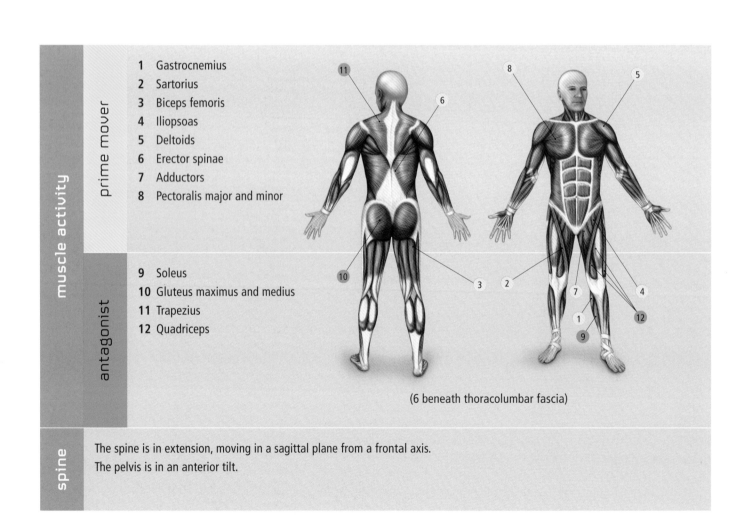

**muscle activity**

**prime mover**

1  Gastrocnemius
2  Sartorius
3  Biceps femoris
4  Iliopsoas
5  Deltoids
6  Erector spinae
7  Adductors
8  Pectoralis major and minor

**antagonist**

9  Soleus
10 Gluteus maximus and medius
11 Trapezius
12 Quadriceps

(6 beneath thoracolumbar fascia)

**spine**

The spine is in extension, moving in a sagittal plane from a frontal axis.
The pelvis is in an anterior tilt.

# Anatomy of the pose

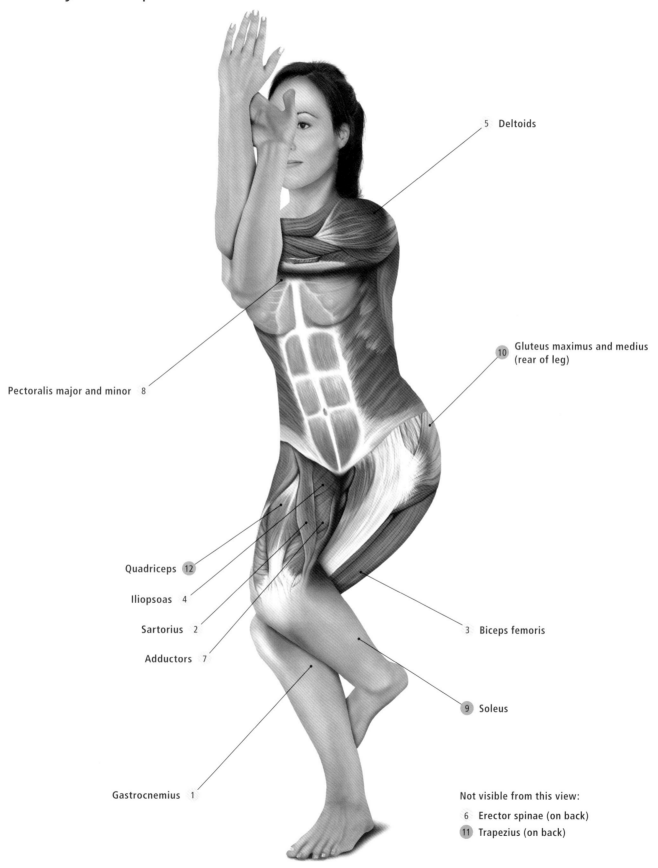

5   Deltoids

10   Gluteus maximus and medius
(rear of leg)

Pectoralis major and minor   8

Quadriceps   12

Iliopsoas   4

Sartorius   2

Adductors   7

3   Biceps femoris

9   Soleus

Gastrocnemius   1

Not visible from this view:

6   Erector spinae (on back)

11   Trapezius (on back)

# Dancer's Pose

## Natarajasana

Dancer's Pose is an energising asana that requires complete mental focus. It is a strong balancing asana that uses every muscle group in the body, and it is considered a backbending asana due to the deep extension of the spine. Overall benefits of Dancer's Pose include increased circulation and improved respiratory function, meaning that general stamina is in turn greatly improved.

The standing leg is completely straight and supports the bodyweight, while the other leg kicks back with the knee flexed. This kicking action ensures that the pelvis tilts forwards, and the upper body also moves forwards, with the spine moving into a backbending position. For this action to occur, the right shoulder and right hip have to rotate outwards, creating a deep stretch in these joints. The ankle and knee of the left leg work hard to stabilise the body, improving their strength and stability. As a result of all the major muscle groups working in synergy in this way, core stability is also greatly improved.

## Level

Intermediate

## Benefits

Dancer's Pose improves stamina. It stretches and strengthens all the major joints, particularly the hips and shoulders, and greatly improves mental focus.

Flexibility of the spine and core stability are also greatly improved.

## Caution

This asana is intensive and should therefore be modified for those with high or low blood pressure.

For practitioners with lower back injuries, there should be minimal rotation in the pelvis to avoid excessive pressure on the spinal discs.

⊕ **Modifications and props**

For blood pressure or lower back issues, modify Dancer's Pose by focusing more on elongating the spine and reaching the left arm upwards, as opposed to extending the spine and left arm forwards.

If it is difficult to bend the knee, place a yoga strap around the ankle and hold the strap with the right hand.

 **Try to**

Elongate the spine, creating a sense of space in the upper body.

Keep the standing leg completely straight to protect the knee joint and improve balance.

Allow the right arm to relax as the right leg kicks back, as this will help the shoulder joint to stretch.

 **Try not to**

Try not to drop the left arm lower than parallel to the floor; instead, keep it on the same level as the eye line and reach forwards strongly.

Avoid rotating the right hip too far, as this may compress the lower back. Instead, allow the right hip to move towards the ground a little.

# How to do it

## ⌃ Step 1

Begin in Mountain Pose (p.54).

## ⌃ Step 2

Rotate the right arm until the inner elbow and palm of the hand are facing outwards. Now transfer the weight to the left leg and bend the right knee, lifting the right foot towards the right gluteal muscle. Place the right hand firmly around the inside of the right ankle. Inhale and extend the left arm directly upwards at the same time, so the left upper arm is in line with the left ear.

## ⌃ Step 3

Press down into the left foot and keep the left leg completely straight by firmly contracting the thigh muscles. Exhale while kicking the right foot back and upwards, so that the upper body tilts forwards, and reach the left arm forwards, too. Breathe evenly as the spine extends forwards. There should be a sense of lifting and length through the upper body.

## ⌃ Step 4

Exhaling, kick the right foot backwards more powerfully, so that the extension of the spine is increased. The right leg should now kick upwards, with the right hip and shoulder turning out to the right. Reach the left arm forwards, keeping the hand in line with the gaze, which should be directly forwards. The chin should be level to the ground.

# Dancer's Pose

## Natarajasana

There are several muscle groups working differently during Dancer's Pose. The hamstrings of the right leg shorten to create the flexion at the knee, while the quadriceps and hip flexors lengthen eccentrically. The posterior deltoid and rotator cuff of the right shoulder externally rotate the right arm. The triceps work concentrically to extend both arms, with the deltoid of the left shoulder contracting isometrically to hold the arm in place, and the pectoral muscles working concentrically to assist. The left leg is fully extended, with the quadriceps contracting concentrically and the hamstrings working to fixate this action. The pelvis is rotated anteriorly and the spine is extended in a backbending position, with the erector spinae shortening concentrically. The latissimus dorsi and rectus abdominis help to fixate the position of the spine.

**muscle activity**

**prime mover**

1 Quadriceps
2 Hamstrings
3 Erector spinae
4 Deltoids
5 Gluteus minimus and maximus

**antagonist**

6 Rectus abdominis
7 Pectoralis major and minor
8 Latissimus dorsi

(3 beneath thoracolumbar fascia)

**spine**

The spine is in extension, moving in a sagittal plane from a frontal axis.
The pelvis is in an anterior tilt position.

# Anatomy of the pose

Deltoids ④

Latissimus dorsi ⑧

Pectoralis major and minor ⑦

Quadriceps ①

Rectus abdominis ⑥

Gluteus minimus and maximus ⑤

Hamstrings ②

**Not visible from this view:**

③ Erector spinae (on back)

# Half Moon Pose

## Ardha Chandrasana

Half Moon Pose is a balancing asana that is very effective in increasing the strength and stability of all the joints, particularly the knees and ankles. Moving into this asana, the spine bends to the right side and the right knee is bent, allowing the right hand to reach the floor just in front of the right foot. As the left foot lifts from the ground, both knees straighten and the legs work powerfully. All four corners of the standing foot are rooted to the ground, while the raised foot is in a neutral position. The spine elongates to create equal length either side of the torso, and the abdominal muscles work hard to support the spine. The arms reach away from the body to create a long line from one hand to the other, stretching the chest and shoulders. The front of the hips and groin also stretch due to the outwards rotation of the left hip. This rotating action should not be forced, however, as it can put unnecessary stress across the lower back joints.

## Level

Intermediate

## Benefits

This pose stretches and strengthens the hips while strengthening the ankle and knee joints. The shoulders and chest are stretched and core stability is greatly improved.

As this asana requires good balance, concentration is also improved.

## Caution

Practitioners with blood pressure issues or lower back injuries, especially spinal disc injuries, should modify this asana.

## ⊕ Modifications and props

If the right leg cannot be straightened when the right hand is on the ground, place a yoga brick under the right hand.

If the spine requires additional support, position the back of the body against a wall.

For neck injuries, keep the gaze directed towards the right hand.

For blood pressure issues, keep the left hand on the left hip.

##  Try to

Contract the leg muscles firmly to help extend the knee joints.

Externally rotate the left side of the body back a little, so the joints are stacked in one line, creating space in the hips and shoulders.

Reach the arms and legs away from the centre of the body to create space in the joints.

##  Try not to

Do not allow the left leg to drop lower than parallel to the floor; instead, create a long straight line from the left heel to the crown of the head.

Try not to drop the left shoulder and left hip forwards; aim to open these joints by drawing the left side of the body backwards.

# How to do it

### ◁ Step 1

Begin in triangle pose (p.62) to the right side. Now place the left hand on the left hip and the right hand on the right lower leg. The left shoulder and left hip should rotate externally, and the neck and crown of the head should lengthen away from the body.

**Step 2 ▷**

Maintain steady breathing while transferring the bodyweight onto the right leg and bend the right knee. Shorten the stance by moving the left foot in a little towards the right. Reach the right hand to the ground just to the side of the foot, in front of the toes. The right hand should now be directly under the right shoulder, and the bodyweight should be mainly on the right leg. The left leg should be straight, with the foot hovering just above the ground.

### ⌃ Step 3

Now straighten the right leg while inhaling and simultaneously raising the left leg parallel to the ground. Extend through the left heel to straighten the left knee, pointing the toes forwards. Contract the thigh muscles firmly and straighten the knees completely.

### ⌃ Step 4

Exhaling, rotate the left hip and left shoulder back slightly to increase the stretch through the left side of the body, before extending the left arm directly upwards. The arms should now create one long line. Keep the neck straight and move the gaze to the left hand.

# Half Moon Pose

## Ardha Chandrasana

Although the spine is laterally flexed to the right in Half Moon Pose, the asana requires equal length through either side of the torso. This initially requires the oblique muscles on the right to contract concentrically as the spine moves into a side-bend. The abdominal muscles, including the rectus abdominis, then work as fixators when the spine begins to elongate. The left oblique muscles contract to externally rotate the left hip and shoulders, moving them into a neutral position, while the quadratus lumborum supports the lumbar spine. The quadriceps work concentrically to extend the knee joints, and the hamstrings lengthen eccentrically to allow this movement. The gluteus maximus helps to extend the hips and the gluteus minimus helps to stabilise the pelvis, while the abductor muscles move the right leg away from the medial line of the body. The standing leg is externally rotated by the quadratus femoris and sartorius hip flexor. The arms are initially externally rotated before being abducted away from the body by the deltoids. The triceps contract concentrically to extend the arms from the elbow joint. The left side of the sternocleidomastoid shortens concentrically to bring the gaze to the left hand.

**muscle activity**

**prime mover**

1 Sternocleidomastoid
2 Quadriceps
3 Gluteus maximus and medius
4 Internal and external obliques
5 Deltoids
6 Quadratus femoris

**antagonist**

7 Hamstrings
8 Quadratus lumborum
9 Sartorius

(6 beneath quadratus femoris; 8 beneath thoracolumbar fascia)

**spine**

The spine is in right lateral flexion, moving in a frontal plane from a sagittal axis.
The pelvis is in a lateral tilt to the right.

# Anatomy of the pose

Not visible from this view:

3 Gluteus maximus and medius (rear of leg)

6 Quadratus femoris (beneath gluteus maximus)

8 Quadratus lumborum (on back)

4 Internal and external obliques

Sternocleidomastoid 1

5 Deltoids

Quadriceps 2

9 Sartorius

7 Hamstrings

# Warrior III Pose

## Virabhadrasana III

Warrior III is considered one of the more challenging balancing poses. Due to the extension of the arms and legs, it requires strength from all the major muscles groups and is therefore very effective at building muscle endurance and aerobic stamina.

Initially, the arms are extended overhead from Mountain Pose, and the spine elongates to create space through the upper body. This action stretches the spine and helps to open the shoulder joints. The thigh muscles, mainly the quadriceps, contract firmly, which helps to extend the knees, while the gluteal muscles extend the hips. This creates a long line from the feet to the hands and stretches all the joints, energising the entire body. When the right leg steps forwards, the spine is lowered parallel to the ground, so the muscles supporting the spine and shoulders have to contract powerfully to maintain the position. The quadriceps and hamstrings work even harder, while the stabilisers of the ankle joints and the abdominal muscles work to maintain the practitioner's balance.

## Level

Intermediate

## Benefits

This asana strengthens the entire body. It stretches the shoulders and gives the practitioner a sense of length through the body.

Because of the intensity of this asana, aerobic and muscle endurance are greatly improved.

## Caution

Because the arms and legs are fully extended, this asana works the lower back intensely and increases the heart rate. This asana should therefore be modified for those with lower back injuries or high or low blood pressure.

## ⊕ Modifications and props

For lower back injuries or blood pressure issues, the arms can be positioned by the side of the body or the hands placed in Prayer Position in front of the sternum.

The alignment of the body can also be modified by moving the spine and raised leg to a diagonal line, as opposed to the lower body being parallel to the ground. This will minimise pressure on the lower back.

## ⊙ Try to

When reaching the arms overhead, try to lengthen and straighten the entire body.

Maintain the straight line through the body and contract the abdominal muscles to support the lumbar region.

The pelvis should be level to the ground when moving into the final position.

## ⊗ Try not to

Try not to lift the shoulders upwards; focus on moving the shoulder blades down, away from the ears.

Avoid rotating the pelvis and instead focus on maintaining a neutral alignment of the hips.

Avoid rounding the spine and instead maintain a straight line through the body, keeping the arms in line with the ears.

# How to do it

**Step 1** ⊗

Begin in Mountain Pose (p.54).

⊗ **Step 2**

Reach the arms out to either side and then extend them up overhead. Interlace the fingers firmly and extend the index fingers, pressing the heels of the hands together firmly. Move the shoulders down, away from the ears. Now press the legs firmly together and elongate the entire body, stretching the back muscles and shoulders. Draw the lower front ribcage in and draw the coccyx down towards the ground.

⊗ **Step 3**

Step the right leg forwards approximately 60 centimetres and transfer the bodyweight to the right leg. Then, keeping the left leg straight, lift the left foot from the ground and extend the left leg backwards as the spine and arms extend forwards. The left leg, spine, and the arms should now create a long diagonal line.

**Step 4** ⊗

Keep the knees straight and contract the thigh and gluteal muscles firmly. Extend into the left heel and point the toes downwards while keeping the hips parallel to the ground. The spine and arms should reach forwards, with the crown of the head pointing forwards, creating a long, straight line from the left heel to the fingertips. Lower the gaze to the ground without dropping the head down.

# Warrior III Pose

## Virabhadrasana III

In Warrior III, the deltoids extend the arms overhead. The arms are internally rotated by the teres major and pectoral muscles and held in place by the serratus anterior. The triceps contract concentrically to extend the elbow joints. The scapulae are initially rotated, before the trapezius muscles move the scapulae down and away from the head. The spine is extended and supported by the erector spinae, quadratus lumborum, and latissimus dorsi. The rectus abdominis isometrically contracts to fixate the spine. The right hip is flexed due to a concentric shortening of the hip flexors, while the left hip joint is extended by the gluteus maximus and the knees are extended by the quadriceps. Both of these muscle groups are in a concentric contraction. The tibialis anterior muscles shorten, and the soleus and gastrocnemius muscles lengthen, to create a dorsiflexion at the ankles.

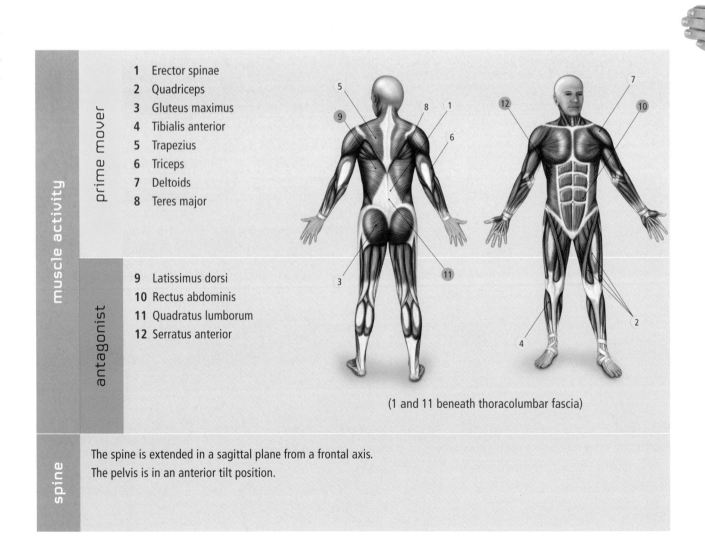

**muscle activity**

**prime mover**

| 1 | Erector spinae |
| 2 | Quadriceps |
| 3 | Gluteus maximus |
| 4 | Tibialis anterior |
| 5 | Trapezius |
| 6 | Triceps |
| 7 | Deltoids |
| 8 | Teres major |

**antagonist**

| 9 | Latissimus dorsi |
| 10 | Rectus abdominis |
| 11 | Quadratus lumborum |
| 12 | Serratus anterior |

(1 and 11 beneath thoracolumbar fascia)

**spine**

The spine is extended in a sagittal plane from a frontal axis.
The pelvis is in an anterior tilt position.

# Anatomy of the pose

5 Trapezius

Teres
8 major

1 Erector spinae (beneath
thoracolumbar fascia)

3 Gluteus
maximus

Triceps 6

Deltoids 7

Latissimus dorsi 9

Serratus anterior 12

Rectus abdominis 10

Quadratus lumborum 11
(beneath thoracolumbar fascia)

Quadriceps 2

Tibialis anterior 4

# Standing Forward Bends

Forward bends, when practised from a standing position, are effective in stretching the whole spine, especially the lower back area. They also stretch the back of the hips and legs, and so are very beneficial for those who partake in sports that tighten these areas, such as running and cycling. They also help to improve posture by lengthening the muscles that surround the spine and back of the pelvis.

On a mental level, forward bends have a calming effect and encourage inward reflection, leading to a decrease in anxiety and an increase in mental well-being.

Wide-legged Forward Bend ............................................... 114
Intense Side Stretch ........................................................... 118

# Standing Forward Bend

## Uttanasana

The Standing Forward Bend is a calming, therapeutic forward bend that can be performed by beginners and advanced yoga practitioners alike, either as a stand-alone pose or as part of a sequence. The forward bend occurs as the hip flexors shorten and the gluteal muscles and hamstrings lengthen, allowing the upper body to hinge forwards. As the upper body moves towards the lower body, the crown of the head moves towards the ground, and the back and neck muscles relax as the spine lengthens, helping to minimise lower back pain. With the head in this position, the brain is calmed and the heart rate automatically slows down, which has a therapeutic effect on the nervous system. The arms are relaxed and the hands press lightly into the ground, which encourages the spine to extend further. The upper back muscles, mainly the trapezius, gently contract to draw the shoulders away from the head. The legs are straight, with the bodyweight distributed evenly through the feet. The calf muscles can be stretched further by keeping the heels on the floor and transferring the weight slightly into the balls of the feet.

## Level

Intermediate

## Benefits

Standing Forward Bend is a calming asana that stretches the lower back and hamstrings and improves the function of the digestive system.

It can relieve pain in the lower back and is known for reducing stress, headaches, and fatigue.

## Caution

Practitioners with low blood pressure, or hamstring or lower back injuries, should be cautious when practising this asana.

### ⊕ Modifications and props

Place the feet hip-width apart to make balancing easier.

To relieve pressure in the lower back, or if the hamstrings are injured, bend the knees.

If the hands do not reach the ground, place them on yoga bricks.

For excessive tension in the neck, a yoga brick can also be placed under the crown of the head to provide additional support.

###  Try to

To lengthen from the lumbar spine, try to tilt the pelvis forwards so the coccyx draws upwards.

Relax the upper body, especially the neck, and allow it to lengthen towards the ground.

Maintain even weight distribution through the feet to avoid stress on the knees and lower back.

###  Try not to

Avoid sinking the bodyweight back into the heels.

Try not to allow the shoulders to lift up around the head, as this will create tension around the neck. Instead, lift them away from the head.

# How to do it

### ⊙ Step 1

Begin in Mountain Pose (p.54).

### Step 2 ⊙

Ensure that the bodyweight is distributed evenly through the feet and place the hands on the hips. Inhale and stretch the spine upwards, so a sense of length is created around the lower back and the crown of the head feels as though it is being drawn gently upwards.

### ⊙ Step 3

Keeping the spine straight and the hands on the hips, breathe out deeply while extending the spine forwards from the waist, moving the upper body towards the legs. The pelvis should tilt forwards and the spine should be elongated. Keep the legs straight and the toes relaxed, and maintain the weight evenly through the soles of the feet.

### ⊙ Step 4

Breathe steadily and, with the upper body pressing lightly on the front of the legs, rest the hands on the ground at either side of the feet. The fingers should be pointing forwards and the elbows pointing backwards. Press lightly into the hands to lengthen the spine further. Now relax the neck completely and gently lift the shoulders away from the head to create a sense of space around the neck.

# Standing Forward Bend

## Uttanasana

The forwards tilt of the pelvis in Standing Forward Bend occurs when the hip flexors, mainly the iliopsoas and rectus femoris, shorten via a concentric contraction. To allow the hips to tilt forwards, the gluteus maximus and hamstrings have to lengthen eccentrically, and the gastrocnemius also lengthens when the legs straighten fully. The extensors of the spine, largely the erector spinae, relax and elongate eccentrically. The abdominal muscles isometrically contract to support the lumbar region, while the trapezius muscles contract concentrically, moving the scapulae away from the head.

**muscle activity**

**prime mover**

| 1 | Iliopsoas |
| 2 | Quadriceps |
| 3 | Rectus femoris |
| 4 | Trapezius |

**antagonist**

| 5 | Hamstrings |
| 6 | Erector spinae |
| 7 | Gluteus maximus |
| 8 | Gastrocnemius |

(6 beneath thoracolumbar fascia)

**spine**

The spine is in forwards flexion, in a sagittal plane.
The pelvis is in an anterior tilt.

# Anatomy of the pose

Erector spinae
(beneath thoracolumbar fascia) 6

7 Gluteus maximus

Trapezius 4

2 Quadriceps

3 Rectus femoris

5 Hamstrings

8 Gastrocnemius

**Not visible from this view:**

1 Iliopsoas (inside hip area)

# Wide-legged Forward Bend

## Prasarita Padottanasana

The Wide-legged Forward Bend is very effective in improving the overall flexibility of the legs and lower back, which can in turn make other asanas, such as Triangle Pose and Extended Side-angle Pose, more achievable. This asana is therapeutic for the spine because the lengthening action of the upper body decompresses the vertebral discs and reduces tension by stretching the back muscles. This effect is initiated by a forwards tilt of the pelvis, which occurs when the hamstrings and gluteus maximus muscles lengthen and the hip flexors shorten. The hips then tip forwards, moving the spine into a forward-flexed position, lengthening all of the lower back muscles. The wide-legged stance also stretches the inner thighs, adductor muscles, and the outer ankles. The hands press into the ground with the elbows bent, which encourages the spine to lengthen further, and the back muscles relax even further, moving the head closer to the ground. The shoulder blades move away from the head as the muscles of the upper back gently contract, which helps to relax the neck.

## Level

Intermediate

## Benefits

This asana can relieve lower back pain and greatly increases the flexibility of the hamstrings and adductor muscles.

Forward bends can also be effective at reducing fatigue and improving sleep patterns.

## Caution

Practitioners with lower back injuries, or groin or hamstring strains, should be cautious when practising this pose.

Deep forward bends can also affect blood pressure, so those with blood pressure issues should be careful not to overexert themselves.

## ⊕ Modifications and props

If the lower back is injured, bend the knees a little to reduce any pressure in the lumbar region.

For groin strains, make the stance shorter.

For low blood pressure, only hold this asana for up to ten breaths.

If it is not possible to reach the ground, place yoga bricks underneath the hands.

##  Try to

Lengthen the spine by drawing the tail bone upwards and the crown of the head downwards.

Create a strong foundation by pressing the feet firmly into the ground, so the feet and legs work more strongly.

Place the hands so that they are in line with the feet.

## ⊗ Try not to

Avoid taking the legs so wide that the asana is no longer stable.

Try not to drop the shoulders around the head. Instead, press firmly into the hands so the elbows move backwards between the legs and the scapulae move down, away from the head.

# How to do it

### ◁ Step 1

Begin in Mountain Pose (p.54).

### ◁ Step 2

Step the feet wide apart while exhaling. Extend the arms out to either side so that they are parallel to the ground. The feet should be aligned directly under the wrists, with the toes pointing forwards.

### ◁ Step 3

Turn the feet inwards slightly and lift the inner arches by pressing down firmly into the outer edges of the feet. Inhaling, contract the thigh muscles and then lengthen the spine upwards. Rest the hands on the hips.

### ⌃ Step 4

Exhale slowly as the upper body folds forwards from the hips, keeping the spine straight and the shoulders drawing back, away from the head. Pause when the spine is parallel to the ground and place the hands on the floor, aligned directly underneath the shoulders, with the arms straight. Inhale and press the sitting bones backwards as the spine lengthens forwards. Rest the gaze on the ground.

### ⌃ Step 5

Exhale and fold more deeply from the lower back, so that the head moves towards the ground. Place the hands in line with the feet. The elbows should point back between the legs, with the forearms perpendicular to the floor and the upper arms parallel to the floor. Keep the legs straight, relax the neck and lengthen through the entire spine.

# Wide-legged Forward Bend

## Prasarita Padottanasana

In this pose, the gluteus minimus and medius muscles contract concentrically and the adductors eccentrically contract, separating the legs away from the medial line of the body, creating a wide stance. The outer edges of the feet then press down into the ground as the peroneus longus lengthens eccentrically and the inner arches of the feet lift a little; this lift is maintained by the tibialis posterior and anterior. The forwards flexion of the spine is due to a concentric shortening of the Iliopsoas and rectus femoris hip flexor muscles, and an eccentric lengthening of the hamstrings, gluteus maximus, erector spinae, soleus, and gastrocnemius. The trapezius muscles contract concentrically to lift the scapulae away from the ears, and the biceps brachii shorten to flex the elbow joints.

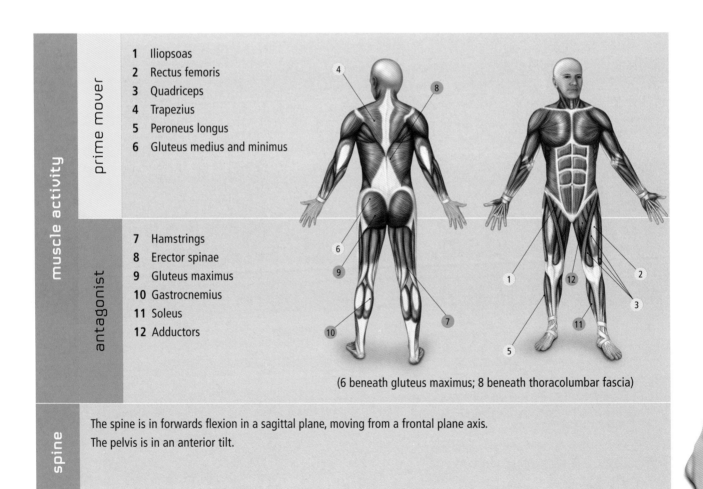

**muscle activity**

**prime mover**

1  Iliopsoas
2  Rectus femoris
3  Quadriceps
4  Trapezius
5  Peroneus longus
6  Gluteus medius and minimus

**antagonist**

7  Hamstrings
8  Erector spinae
9  Gluteus maximus
10  Gastrocnemius
11  Soleus
12  Adductors

(6 beneath gluteus maximus; 8 beneath thoracolumbar fascia)

**spine**

The spine is in forwards flexion in a sagittal plane, moving from a frontal plane axis.
The pelvis is in an anterior tilt.

# Anatomy of the pose

Not visible from this view:

1  Iliopsoas (inside hip area, deep)
7  Hamstrings (rear of thigh)

9  Gluteus maximus

Gluteus medius and maximus
(beneath gluteus maximus)  6

8  Erector spinae (beneath thoracolumbar fascia)

Adductors  12

Rectus femoris  2

Quadriceps  3

10  Gastrocnemius

5  Peroneus longus

11  Soleus

4  Trapezius

# Intense Side Stretch

## Parsvottanasana

Intense Side Stretch is a deep stretch for the hamstrings, calf muscles, back of the hips, and lower back. It aims to create space along the spine and through the upper body. The spine bends from the pelvis, which tilts forwards, and moves towards the right leg. This creates a strong stretch through the hamstrings and gluteal muscles, which lengthen, and a contraction through the hip flexors. The heels are aligned in a straight line, which means this posture requires a good balance and the practitioner's complete focus. The small stabilising muscles of the ankles have to contract to maintain this alignment of the ankle joints. The arms are in Reverse Prayer Position, with the hands behind the back, which helps to open and stretch the chest and front of the shoulders. By pressing the hands together in this way, the wrist flexors stretch and the upper back muscles contract and draw the shoulder blades towards one another, opening the shoulders further.

## Level

Intermediate

## Benefits

This asana stretches the lower body, especially the hamstrings and gluteal and calf muscles, and opens the chest and front of the shoulders.

It improves balance and mental focus and also stability of the ankle joints.

## Caution

Practitioners with wrist, ankle, or lower back injuries should modify this asana.

Forward bends can affect blood pressure, so again, those with blood pressure issues shouldcaution should be taken when practising this pose.

## ⊕ Modifications and props

If it is not possible to place the hands behind the back, fold the arms behind the back and hold either elbow instead, drawing the scapulae towards one another to keep the front of the shoulders open.

For lower back issues, bend the knee of the front leg a little.

For ankle injuries, position the feet diagonally, as this will make balancing easier.

## ⊘ Try to

Before folding forwards, align the right side of the pelvis with the left side, so it is in a neutral position, and stretch the spine upwards.

Contract the thigh muscles and spread out the toes to improve balance.

## ⊗ Try not to

Try not to round the spine when folding forwards; instead, focus on elongating the spine from the lower back to the neck.

Try not to let the right hip move forwards. Focus on moving it back, so it remains in line with the left hip.

Do not lift the head when in the final phase of the asana. Let the neck relax, with the gaze resting on the middle of the lower leg.

# How to do it

### ⊘ Step 1

Begin in Mountain Pose (p.54).

### ⊘ Step 2

On an exhale, step the feet approximately 1 metre apart. Exhale and turn the right foot out ninety degrees and the left foot in forty-five degrees. Now turn the entire body ninety degrees to the right, so the right leg is in front and the left leg is behind. The legs and spine should be straight, with the arms resting by the side of the body. Press the feet firmly into the ground, contract the thigh muscles, and relax the toes.

### ⊼ Step 3

Now begin to internally rotate the arms from the shoulder joints, so that the palms of the hands face backwards. Bend the elbows and place the backs of the hands onto the middle of the back while exhaling. Press the thumbs together and move the elbows backwards to help stretch the chest area; this is known as 'Reverse Prayer Position'. On an inhale, lift the sternum upwards and lift the chin away from the chest, to create a slight extension of the spine.

### ⊼ Step 4

Exhale deeply and hinge forwards by tilting the pelvis forwards and extending from the lower back. Keep the legs straight as the upper body moves slowly towards the front leg, and keep pressing the hands together. Once the front of the ribcage is resting on the right leg, allow the neck to relax and bring the gaze towards the middle of the right lower leg. Continue to breathe deeply.

# Intense Side Stretch

## Parsvottanasana

For the Reverse Prayer Position of the hands used in this pose, the shoulder rotators inwardly rotate the humerus bones and the biceps brachii shorten, while the triceps lengthen to allow flexion at the elbow. This allows the hands to be positioned behind the middle spine with the wrists extended and the palms together. The anterior deltoids eccentrically stretch while the posterior deltoids and trapezius assist in drawing the scapulae together, creating a stretch across the chest. The quadriceps are concentrically contracted, extending the knee joints, while the sartorius hip flexor muscle, and other hip external rotators, externally rotates the left leg. The forwards flexion of the spine is caused initially by a concentric shortening of the iliopsoas, resulting in a forwards tilt of the pelvis. The erector spinae, quadratus lumborum, and hamstrings lengthen eccentrically to allow this movement.

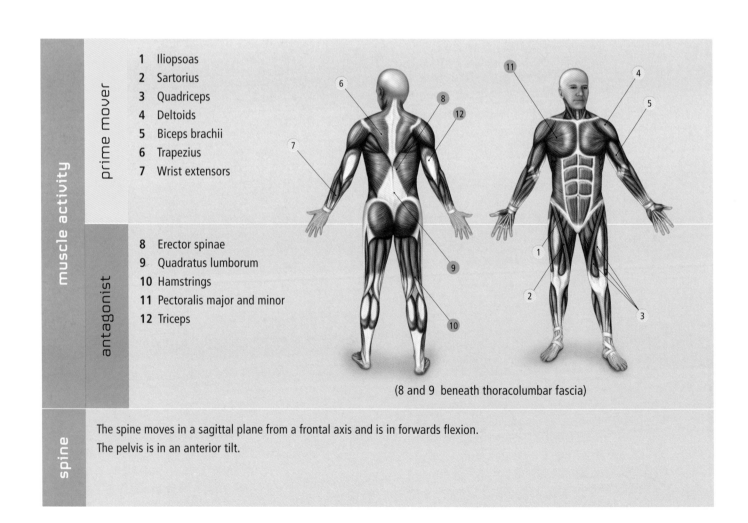

**muscle activity**

**prime mover**

1  Iliopsoas
2  Sartorius
3  Quadriceps
4  Deltoids
5  Biceps brachii
6  Trapezius
7  Wrist extensors

**antagonist**

8  Erector spinae
9  Quadratus lumborum
10  Hamstrings
11  Pectoralis major and minor
12  Triceps

(8 and 9  beneath thoracolumbar fascia)

**spine**

The spine moves in a sagittal plane from a frontal axis and is in forwards flexion.
The pelvis is in an anterior tilt.

# Anatomy of the pose

**Not visible from this view:**

1 Iliopsoas (inside hip area, deep)

9 Quadratus lumborum   (8 and 9 beneath thoracolumbar fascia)

8 Erector spinae

6 Trapezius

7 Wrist extensors (not visible)

5 Biceps brachii (not visible)

2 Sartorius

12 Triceps

10 Hamstrings

4 Deltoids

3 Quadriceps

Pectoralis major and minor 11

# Seated Poses

Seated yoga asanas may involve twists, forward bends, or simply sitting with the spine straight, and are mainly practised after a standing yoga sequence. They are generally less demanding than standing asanas as fewer muscle groups are utilised, but they can be more challenging mentally for some practitioners as the body needs to remain still. In this way, seated yoga postures can be used for quiet contemplation and are also useful for some people with limited mobility. Some seated yoga asanas in which the spine remains straight are also useful when practising pranayama, because the lungs are not compressed in any way.

# Seated Forward Bend

## Paschimottanasana

The Seated Forward Bend is an effective stretch for the hamstrings, calf muscles, and lower back. The pelvis tilts forwards and the spine extends forwards, encouraging the bodyweight to move onto the front part of the sitting bones, which then increases the stretch in the hamstrings and lower back. The legs are fully extended from the knee joint, with the quadriceps contracting and helping to press the legs together. The hands are positioned around the outer edges of the feet, helping to stretch the calf muscles further. The position of the feet also helps to lengthen the Achilles tendon and the ligaments of the ankle joint. The shoulders draw down, away from the head, which gives a sense of length in the upper back and neck. By stretching the spine and back of the legs like this, postural alignment is improved, because it becomes easier to straighten the spine when standing. By lowering the upper body and head, the heart rate is reduced, helping to calm the nervous system and, therefore, the mind.

**Level**

Beginner

**Benefits**

The Seated Forward Bend stretches the back of the legs and lumbar region and creates a sense of length through the entire body.

As the abdomen rests on the thighs, this asana also helps to stimulate digestion.

**Caution**

If the lower back is injured, which includes injuries to the spinal discs, extra care should be taken when practising this asana.

If the hamstrings or calf muscles are strained, the knees should be slightly bent.

⊕ **Modifications and props**

If it is not possible to straighten the spine, place a yoga block directly underneath the sitting bones. This will encourage a more neutral alignment.

If the lower back is injured, bend the knees a little and place a rolled-up yoga mat behind the knees to support them.

If the feet cannot be reached, a yoga strap can be used.

 **Try to**

Maintain length through the spine and draw the shoulders down, away from the head, so that the neck also lengthens.

Maintain a sense of strength through the lower body by contracting the thigh muscles, pressing into the heels and keeping the toes pointing upwards.

 **Try not to**

Try not to round the spine and avoid lifting the shoulders towards the head. Instead, focus on elongating the spine from the lower back by tilting the pelvis forwards.

Avoid pulling on the feet very strongly as this may cause strain.

Do not look directly forwards as this might strain the neck; instead, rest the gaze on the lower legs.

# How to do it

**Step 1** ⊘

Begin in Staff Pose (p.54).

**Step 2** ⊘

Inhale while extending the arms directly upwards in line with the ears. Keep the shoulders drawing down away from the head. Press into the heels and flex the feet, pointing the toes directly upwards.

**Step 3** ⊘

Keeping the arms in line with the ears, begin to exhale and, at the same time, tilt the pelvis forwards so that the spine extends forwards. Contract the abdominal muscles to support the lower back and maintain the strength through the legs.

⊘ **Step 4**

Now lower the hands to the outside edges of the feet and slowly fold forwards. On an exhale, bring the front of the upper body to rest on the legs. The elbows should point out to either side and the hands should gently pull on the outside edges of the feet to help lengthen the spine and the stretch through the back of the legs. Move the crown of the head towards the feet and relax the neck, resting the gaze on the lower legs. Continue to breathe deeply.

# Seated Forward Bend

## Paschimottanasana

In this pose, the quadriceps contract concentrically, while the hamstrings lengthen eccentrically, resulting in full extension of the knee joints. The tibialis anterior contract concentrically, creating dorsiflexion of the ankle. This then eccentrically lengthens the hamstrings, soleus, and gastrocnemius, with the stretch increased further when moving into the full asana. The pelvis tilts forwards when the iliopsoas shortens, creating a forwards flexion at the lumbar spine. The gluteus maximus and erector spinae then lengthen eccentrically, allowing the spine to fold forwards. The scapulae are drawn down, away from the head, when the trapezius and serratus anterior muscles contract concentrically.

**muscle activity**

**prime mover**

1 Iliopsoas
2 Quadriceps
3 Serratus anterior
4 Tibialis anterior
5 Trapezius

**antagonist**

6 Hamstrings
7 Erector spinae
8 Gluteus maximus
9 Soleus and gastrocnemius

(7 beneath thoracolumbar fascia)

**spine**

The spine moves in a sagittal plane from a frontal axis and is in forwards flexion.
The pelvis is in an anterior tilt.

# Anatomy of the pose

**Not visible from this view:**

1  Iliopsoas (inside hip area, deep)
4  Tibialis anterior (lower leg)
9  Soleus and gastrocnemius (lower leg)

6  Hamstrings
5  Trapezius
2  Quadriceps
3  Serratus anterior
7  Erector spinae
(beneath thoracolumbar fascia)
8  Gluteus maximus

# Boat Pose

## Navasana

Boat Pose is an intense asana that requires considerable strength of the abdominal, lower back, and leg muscles. To hold the spine in position, the abdominal and lower back muscles contract, supporting the lumbar region. The legs are fully extended and raised from the ground by a strong contraction of the iliopsoas, quadriceps, and hip flexors. The triceps muscles shorten to straighten the arms and hold them parallel to the floor, and the shoulder blades draw together and down, away from the ears. This action helps the sternum lift upwards slightly, encouraging a sense of lift and length from the lower back, and ensuring the core muscles work even harder. Regular practice of Boat Pose helps overall strength and endurance, especially of the core muscles. This, in turn, helps improve the performance of other asanas that require a good deal of core stability, such as Headstand Pose. As the iliopsoas and hip flexors shorten in Boat Pose, it is useful to follow this asana with a hip-opening pose, such as Cobbler's Pose or Pigeon Pose, to stretch these muscles.

## Level

Intermediate

## Benefits

Boat Pose significantly increases the strength of the lower back and abdominal area. The muscles that support the pelvis – the iliopsoas – also strengthen, as they help to move the legs closer to the torso. Mental focus is also improved.

## Caution

Boat Pose works the lower back hard, so people with lower back injuries should modify this asana. Those with hernias should not practise Boat Pose.

### ⊕ Modifications and props

To minimise pressure on the lower back, bend the knees so that the lower legs are level to the floor. For additional support, hold the backs of the thighs. This will make it easier to lift the sternum and stop the spine from rounding.

### ⊘ Try to

Contract the abdominal muscles to support the lower back area. Aim to lift the sternum upwards and move the shoulder blades towards one another, so the lower back does not curve and excessive pressure is not put on the lumbar spine.

Try to press the legs together firmly, so all the muscles of the legs are working.

### ⊗ Try not to

Try not to round the spine, as this may put pressure on the lower back.

Avoid lowering the legs to a point where there is strain on the hip flexors. Instead, focus on maintaining the neutral alignment of the spine and keep the feet in line with the gaze.

# How to do it

**Step 1** ⊗

Begin in Staff Pose (p.54).

**Step 2** ⊗

Bend the legs so that the feet are flat on the floor and there is approximately 0.5 metres between the sitting bones and the heels. Place the hands lightly around the backs of the thighs. Transfer the bodyweight towards the back of the pelvis and lean the spine back slightly, keeping it in a straight line. Contract the abdominal muscles so the spine is supported. Breathe evenly throughout.

⊗ **Step 3**

Inhale while lifting the feet so that the lower legs are parallel to the ground. Press the legs together and extend the arms forwards so that they are also parallel to the ground. The palms should be facing towards one another. Continue to breathe steadily and move the shoulder blades towards one another, so the chest lifts a little. The chin should be level to the floor.

**Step 4** ⊗

Now, on an exhale, fully extend the legs, contracting the muscles of the legs strongly and pressing the legs together more firmly. Keep the chest lifted and the arms level to the ground. The abdominal muscles will need to work harder now and should be drawn in towards the spine. Breathe steadily throughout.

# Boat Pose

## Navasana

In Boat Pose, the hip flexors, mainly the iliopsoas, are concentrically shortened, moving the legs towards the torso and the hips into a partially flexed position. The pelvis is tilted back so the majority of the bodyweight is on the coccyx and ischium bones. The spine is in a slightly extended position and angled backwards, so that the spine and legs make a 'V' shape.

To support the position of the spine, the rectus and transversus abdominis work powerfully as fixators, as do the erector spinae and latissimus dorsi. The quadriceps and soleus concentrically contract to fully extend the legs and ankles, as do the triceps, to extend the arms from the elbow joints. The anterior deltoids fixate the arms in place and the posterior deltoids hold the scapulae in place.

**muscle activity**

**prime mover**

| 1 | Rectus abdominis |
|---|---|
| 2 | Iliopsoas |
| 3 | Triceps |
| 4 | Deltoids |
| 5 | Erector spinae |
| 6 | Quadriceps |
| 7 | Soleus |

**antagonist**

| 8 | Transversus abdominis |
|---|---|
| 9 | Latissimus dorsi |
| 10 | Hamstrings |
| 11 | Biceps brachii |
| 12 | Tibialis anterior |

(5 beneath thoracolumbar fascia)

**spine**

The spine is in a neutral position, moving in a sagittal plane from a frontal axis.

The pelvis is in an anterior tilt position.

# Anatomy of the pose

**Not visible from this view:**

2   Iliopsoas (inside hip area, deep)

12  Tibialis anterior

7   Soleus

Biceps brachii  11

Deltoids  4

Triceps  3

9  Latissimus dorsi

Erector spinae
5  (beneath thoracolumbar fascia)

1  Rectus abdominis

Hamstrings 10

8  Transversus abdominis

Quadriceps  6

# Half Lord of the Fishes Pose

## Ardha Matsyendrasana

Half Lord of the Fishes is a therapeutic spinal twist that increases the flexibility of the spine. The rotating action stretches the upper body on one side and compresses the other. On the compressed side, the internal organs are gently massaged, which is thought to have a detoxifying effect, especially on the digestive system.

The oblique abdominal muscles stretch on one side and lengthen on the other, while both sides of the back stretch and lengthen. The right arm is extended and supports the torso, while the left arm acts as a lever against the right leg to increase the rotation of the spine. The legs are bent, with the right foot pressing down into the ground, which encourages the spine to extend upwards, and the left leg is relaxed on the floor. This position of the legs helps to stretch the hips and gluteal muscles, which in turn can help alleviate lower backache. The overall effect of this asana is a gentle stretch into the hips and shoulders and a strong stretch of the back muscles.

## Level

Intermediate

## Benefits

This asana increases the spine's flexibility by stretching the back muscles and connective tissues of the ribcage. It also stretches the hips.

The twisting action of the upper body gently stimulates the internal organs, which improves their general functioning.

## Caution

This twisting action is not appropriate for spinal disc injuries or injuries to the neck.

Those with conditions affecting the knee joint may need to modify the position of the legs.

### ⊕ Modifications and props

If the spine is rounded, place a yoga block underneath the hips. This will help to bring the pelvis and lower back into a more neutral alignment.

If the knees are injured, keep the left leg straight and move the right foot away from the hips a little.

###  Try to

Elongate the spine by extending it upwards before twisting. Press the right foot into the ground to assist with this action.

For a deeper twist, press the left arm against the right outer thigh more firmly, but not to the point of overexertion.

### ⊗ Try not to

Avoid rounding the spine, as this will put undue pressure on the spinal discs.

Don't twist the neck too far; instead, turn the head gently towards the right shoulder.

Avoid pressing the left arm too strongly against the right thigh.

# How to do it

### ◁ Step 1

Begin in Staff Pose (p.54).

### ◁ Step 2

Bend the right knee and place the right foot on the ground next to the outer left hip, so the right leg is positioned over the left thigh. The sole of the right foot should be on the ground with the toes pointing forwards. The spine should remain straight. Ensure the breathing is slow and even.

### Step 3 ▷

Now bend the left leg and place the left foot next to the right outer hip. The left leg should be relaxed, with the entire outer ankle, foot, and right leg resting on the ground. Flex the left foot by moving the left toes towards the left shin, creating flexion in the ankle joint. Press the right foot into the ground to create more lift through the upper body.

### ⌃ Step 4

Place the right hand on the ground behind the back, in line with the coccyx, and extend the left arm directly upwards on an inhale. Feel the lift and lengthen through the entire spine as the upper body rotates towards the right on an exhale. The left shoulder should be moving forwards and the right shoulder moving backwards.

### ⌃ Step 5

On an exhale, bend the left elbow and place it firmly against the outer right thigh. The fingers and thumb of the left hand should be pointing directly upwards and the left arm should pressing firmly against the outer right thigh to increase the rotation of the spine. Keep the chin parallel to the ground and gaze over the right shoulder. Breathe steadily.

# Half Lord of the Fishes Pose

## Ardha Matsyendrasana

In this seated twist, the quadriceps stretch eccentrically to allow the flexion at the knee joints, which is instigated by the hamstrings contracting concentrically. The iliopsoas on the right side contracts concentrically to flex and adduct the right thigh and bring it in towards the upper body. The left side of the hip is externally rotated and the iliopsoas lengthens eccentrically to abduct the leg away from the upper body, so it can rest on the ground. The oblique muscles work on either side of the torso to create the rotation of the thoracic spine and ribcage, with the right side obliques shortening concentrically and the left side obliques lengthening eccentrically. The latissimus dorsi also lengthens and shortens in the same way, and the rectus abdominis works isometrically to support the upper body. The left arm is flexed at the elbow due to the concentric shortening of the biceps brachii, and the right arm is externally rotated and fully extended at the elbow due to the triceps also shortening concentrically.

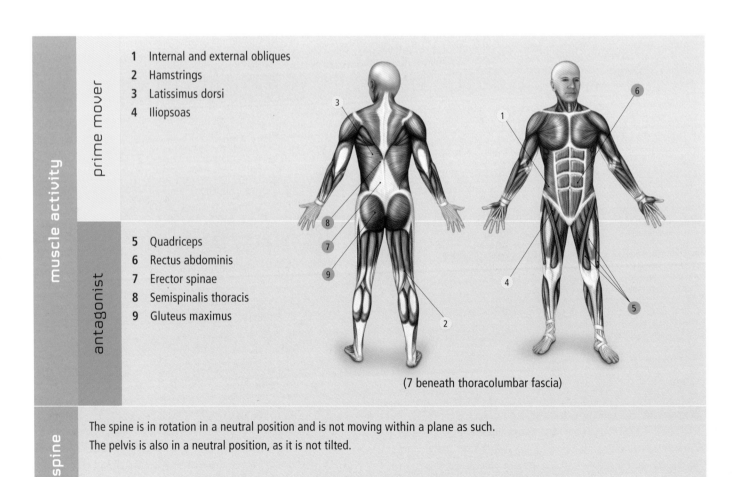

**muscle activity**

**prime mover**

1  Internal and external obliques
2  Hamstrings
3  Latissimus dorsi
4  Iliopsoas

**antagonist**

5  Quadriceps
6  Rectus abdominis
7  Erector spinae
8  Semispinalis thoracis
9  Gluteus maximus

(7 beneath thoracolumbar fascia)

**spine**

The spine is in rotation in a neutral position and is not moving within a plane as such.
The pelvis is also in a neutral position, as it is not tilted.

# Anatomy of the pose

Not visible from this view:

4   Iliopsoas (inside hip area, deep)
7   Erector spinae
8   Semispinalis thoracis

Quadriceps 5

Latissimus dorsi 3

Internal and
external obliques 1

Gluteus maximus 9

6 Rectus abdominis

2   Hamstrings

# Cobbler's Pose

## Baddha Konasana

Cobbler's Pose is a hip-opening asana that improves the flexibility of the hips and stretches the lower back. It aims to stretch the inner thigh muscles and groin, and it is effective for preparing the hips for other hip-opening asanas, such as Pigeon Pose and Dancer's Pose.

The smaller gluteal muscles around the outer hips shorten to move the thigh bones out to either side, which then allows the soles of the feet come together. This action not only stretches the ankles, but lengthens the inner thigh muscles, and stretches the connective tissue around the knee joints too. The pelvis at this point is in a neutral position. To flex the spine forwards over the ankles and feet, the spine moves into a forwards-tilt position. This greatly intensifies the stretch in the inner thigh and groin, and the lower back and back of the gluteal muscles are also stretched. The hands are placed around the feet and the arms are bent with the elbows resting on the inner legs, which helps to stretch the inner thighs and hips further.

## Level

Intermediate

## Benefits

Cobbler's Pose opens the hips and stretches the inner thighs. It can help to alleviate lower backache and has been known to alleviate sciatica.

## Caution

For those with either groin or knee injuries, caution should be taken when practising Cobbler's Pose.

For practitioners with lower back injuries, such as a herniated vertebral disc, the forwards bend part of this asana should not be practised.

## ⊕ Modifications and props

If the hips are very inflexible, remain in an upright position and allow the legs to relax without bending forwards.

To take pressure off the knees, move the feet further away from the pelvis.

If the pelvis is tilting backwards, place a yoga block underneath the pelvis to bring it into a neutral alignment.

##  Try to

Focus on lifting the spine upwards and allow the legs to relax towards the ground slowly, so the front of the hips open gradually.

When folding the upper body forwards, the spine should remain elongated.

The elbows can press onto the inner thighs to increase the stretch of the hips, but avoid this adjustment if the hips are very inflexible.

##  Try not to

Try not to round the spine. Instead, lengthen the spine upwards and lift the sternum a little, and maintain the length through the upper body when folding forwards.

To avoid tension in the shoulders and neck area, keep the shoulders down, away from the head.

# How to do it

**Step 1** ⊘

Begin in Staff Pose (p.54).

**Step 2** ⊘

Bend the knees until the heels are a few centimetres away from the pelvis and bring the soles of the feet together. Now exhale while letting the legs drop to either side, moving them towards the ground. Move the heels as close to the pelvis as you can without feeling pressure in the knees, and place the hands around the feet with the fingers interlaced. Keep the spine upright and straight. Now inhale and at the same time lift the sternum a little, drawing the shoulders down away from the head. Press the feet together and allow the legs to move closer to the ground by relaxing the hips.

⊘ **Step 3**

Now exhale slowly while the pelvis tilts forwards and the upper body extends forwards. The chest should move towards the feet and the stretch of the inner thighs should increase. Rest the elbows on the inner legs. Keep breathing deeply as the head and neck relax, and rest the gaze on the toes.

# Cobbler's Pose

## Baddha Konasana

The quadriceps are eccentrically lengthened and the hamstrings are concentrically contracted, fully flexing the knees. The piriformis, sartorius, and gluteus medius and minimus all work in unison and contract concentrically to externally rotate the femurs, allowing the soles of the feet to press together and the legs to rest on the floor. In this position, the adductors stretch eccentrically. The pelvis is in an anterior tilt position, and quadratus lumborum and erector spinae stretch eccentrically to allow the spine to flex forwards over the ankles and feet. The trapezius muscles move the scapulae away from the head and the biceps brachii shorten concentrically to flex the elbows.

**muscle activity**

**prime mover**

1  Gluteus medius and minimus
2  Sartorius
3  Trapezius
4  Piriformis
5  Hamstrings
6  Biceps brachii

**antagonist**

7  Adductors
8  Erector spinae
9  Quadratus lumborum

(1 and 4 beneath gluteus maximus; 8 and 9 beneath thoracolumbar fascia)

**spine**

The spine moves in a sagittal plane from a frontal axis and is in forwards flexion.
The pelvis is in an anterior tilt position.

# Anatomy of the pose

**Not visible from this view:**

1 Piriformis (beneath gluteus maximus)

4 Gluteus medius and minimus (beneath gluteus maximus)

6 Erector spinae (on back)

8 Biceps brachii

3 Trapezius

5 Hamstrings

7 Adductors (inner thigh)

9 Quadratus lumborum (beneath thoracolumbar fascia)

2 Sartorius

# Backbend Poses

Backbending asanas extend the spine in the opposite direction to forward bends and are generally practised towards the end of a hatha yoga session, when the body is warm and more flexible. They are effective in stretching the abdominal muscles and the hip flexors. In more advanced backbending asanas, such as Wheel Pose, the entire front of the body, including the shoulders and chest area, is also deeply stretched. This has a dramatic effect in improving overall flexibility.

Mentally, backbends are invigorating, leading to clarity of mind and increased energy levels within the body.

# Cobra Pose

## Bhujangasana

Cobra Pose is one of the gentler backbending asanas that strengthens the entire spine. The arms are in a flexed position and, as the hands press lightly into the ground and the chest lifts from the floor, the extensor muscles of the spine shorten and move into an extended position, which increases the flexibility of the thoracic spine in particular.

The muscles of the upper back, including the trapezius muscles, move the shoulder blades away from the head, allowing the neck to elongate, so the entire upper body feels lengthened. The feet are stretched away from the body and press into the floor, which helps the thigh and gluteal muscles to contract. At the same time, the abdominal muscles lengthen and stretch, and the light pressure on the lower abdominal area has a therapeutic effect on the digestive system.

## Level

Beginner

## Benefits

Cobra Pose strengthens the legs and extensor muscles of the spine. It also stretches the abdominal and chest muscles.

## Caution

Practitioners with vertebral disc or wrist injuries should be cautious when practising Cobra Pose.

### ⊕ Modifications and props

In the case of back injuries, only lift the top part of the chest from the floor, so the extension of the spine is minimal. Press into the hands more, so that the arms can provide more support to the spine.

For lower back injuries, separate the feet so they are hip-width apart.

For wrist injuries, avoid pressing firmly into the hands.

###  Try to

Maintain a sense of length through the spine and legs.

To create lift, use predominantly the muscles of the back, rather than pressing into the hands and using only the arms.

Actively move the shoulders away from the ears to create space through the neck.

###  Try not to

Avoid lifting the chin beyond horizontal and compressing the back of the neck. Instead, aim to elongate the neck.

Try not to overwork the gluteal muscles by tensing them, as this may put undue tension on the lower back.

# How to do it

⊗ **Step 1**

From lying face down, place the hands on either side of the chest with the fingers and thumbs pointing forwards. Press the legs together with the feet stretching away. Press the tops of the feet into the ground and draw the heels towards one another. Contract the gluteal and thigh muscles. Maintain a steady breath throughout.

**Step 2** ⊗

Now press the arms against the ribcage and press the hands lightly into the ground. Inhale while beginning to lift the chest, as though peeling the sternum away from the ground. Stretch across the chest and move the shoulders away from the ears. Keep the chin level to the floor and the gaze lifted slightly, to maintain length in the neck.

# Cobra Pose

## Bhujangasana

During Cobra Pose the thoracic spine is in an extended position due to a concentric contraction of the erector spinae and latissimus dorsi muscle groups. The elbows are in a flexed position, with the triceps lengthening eccentrically and the biceps brachii shortening concentrically. The triceps then fixate the arms in place via an isometric contraction. The scapulae are moved down, away from the head and towards the spine, by the trapezius and rhomboid muscles. The hip and knee joints are fully extended, with the legs lengthening away from the torso and the tops of the feet pressing into the ground. The quadriceps contract concentrically and gluteus maximus contracts isometrically, providing support for the sacroiliac and pelvic area. As the chest lifts, the pectoral and rectus abdominis muscles lengthen eccentrically, allowing the spine to extend and stretch away from the ground.

## Anatomy of the pose

3  Trapezius
4  Rhomboids (beneath trapezius)
8  Pectoralis major and minor
5  Triceps
9  Rectus abdominis
1  Erector spinae (beneath thoracolumbar fascia
7  Gluteus maximu

**muscle activity**

**prime mover**

1 Erector spinae
2 Quadriceps
3 Trapezius
4 Rhomboids
5 Triceps

**antagonist**

6 Hamstrings
7 Gluteus maximus
8 Pectoralis major and minor
9 Rectus abdominis

(1 beneath thoracolumbar fascia; 4 beneath trapezius)

**spine**

The spine is in an extended position and moves in a sagittal plane from a frontal axis.
The pelvis is in a neutral position.

6 Hamstrings

2 Quadriceps

# Upward-facing Dog Pose

## Urdhva Mukha Svanasana

This asana involves a backbending position and demands considerable strength from the arms and legs. The spine is in an extended position, which lengthens the muscles at the front on the body, particularly the hip flexors and abdominal muscles. The legs are stretched back, with the feet hip-width apart, and the thighs and gluteal muscles work strongly to support the lower back. The abdominal muscles, although stretched, also contract to support the lower back. The arms are extended, with the triceps contracting powerfully and helping to lift the upper body. The chest and front of the shoulders stretch while the muscles of the upper back work to move the shoulder blades downwards. This action opens the whole of the front upper body, which in turn improves postural alignment. The chin is a little above parallel to the ground with the gaze lifted. This helps encourages a lifting action through the crown.

## Level

Intermediate

## Benefits

This asana improves posture by stretching the chest, shoulders, abdomen, and the front of the hips.

It increases the flexibility of the entire spine and energises the body, relieving fatigue.

## Caution

Those with back injuries should be cautious when practising this asana.

Those with conditions such as herniated discs or wrist injuries should not practise Upward-facing Dog Pose. Cobra Pose is more appropriate.

## ⊕ Modifications and props

If it is too challenging to maintain the lift of the hips and legs off the floor, position a rolled-up blanket underneath the tops of the thighs. This will give the lower back more support.

## ⊘ Try to

Really lengthen through the entire spine and aim to create space within the upper body.

Press the feet firmly into the ground so the legs are strong. This will help to avoid pressure in the lower back.

To avoid undue tension in the neck area, try to move the shoulders away from the head and work the upper back to draw the shoulder blades downwards.

## ⊗ Try not to

Avoid 'hanging' from the shoulders. Instead, ensure the arms are strong and the upper body is open.

Try not to relax the legs; instead, keep the leg and gluteal muscles strong to support the spine.

Avoid taking the feet wider than hip-width apart, as this can put stress on the lower back area.

# How to do it

### ⊛ Step 1

Lie face down on the ground and stretch the legs straight back with the tops of the feet resting on the ground. Ensure the breath is even and that the feet are no more than hip-width apart. Now bend the elbows and place the palms of the hands on the ground either side of the upper body, so they align approximately halfway down the ribcage. The forearms should be almost perpendicular to the ground. Spread the fingers and thumbs so the hands feel stretched.

### ⊘ Step 2

Inhale deeply and, on the next exhale, press the hands firmly onto the ground and begin to straighten the arms while simultaneously lifting the torso directly upwards, until the legs and front of the hips also lift a few inches off the ground. The tops of the feet should remain on the ground. Stretch all the way to the toes and firm the legs so the gluteal muscles also contract.

### Step 3 ⊘

Breathing steadily, focus now on pressing the chest forwards a little and drawing the shoulders down until the chest feels more open. As the front of the shoulders stretch, the inner elbows will face forwards. Lift the chin slightly higher than parallel to the ground, maintaining the length through the neck and lifting the gaze upwards at the same time.

# Upward-facing Dog Pose

## Urdhva Mukha Svanasana

In Upward-facing Dog Pose, the triceps are in a concentric contraction and the biceps brachii are lengthened, fully extending the elbows and straightening the arms. As the hands are directly underneath the shoulders, the entire spine then moves into an extended position, with a concentric contraction of the erector spinae and latissimus dorsi muscles. The rectus and transversus abdominis muscles eccentrically contract as the spine extends, and the anterior shoulders and inner elbows externally rotate, while the trapezius moves the scapulae downwards, resulting in the pectoral muscles eccentrically lengthening. The quadriceps are concentrically contracted, extending the knees and straightening the legs. The hamstrings support this action by contracting isometrically, as do the gluteus maximus muscles. This supports the lumbar spine and sacroiliac area.

## Anatomy of the pose

Deltoids  5

3  Trapezius

Pectoralis major and minor  8

1  Erector spinae (beneath thoracolumbar fascia)

7  Gluteus maximus

2  Quadriceps

Triceps  4

6  Hamstrings

Rectus abdominis  9

**muscle activity**

**prime mover**

1 Erector spinae
2 Quadriceps
3 Trapezius
4 Triceps
5 Deltoids

**antagonist**

6 Hamstrings
7 Gluteus maximus
8 Pectoralis major and minor
9 Rectus abdominis

(1 beneath thoracolumbar fascia)

**spine**

The spine is in an extended position and moves in a sagittal plane from a frontal axis.
The pelvis is in a posterior tilt position.

# Pigeon Pose

## Eka Pada Kapotasana

Pigeon Pose is a hip-opening asana that not only stretches the muscles of the pelvis, but prepares the hips for other asanas, such as Dancer's Pose and Cobbler's Pose. The front leg is bent and the angle of the thigh and right knee means that all the gluteal muscles of the right hip are stretched. This has a therapeutic effect on the lumbar region, and with regular practice, Pigeon Pose can ease recurrent lower back pain and sciatica, because it also stretches the muscles around the back of the pelvis.

The left leg is extended behind the body with the hip flexors stretching and lengthening. By extending the left foot away from the body, the ankle joint is stretched. The spine flexes forwards over the right leg with the arms resting on the floor, which helps stretch the upper body. Opening the hips in this way increases the general mobility and flexibility of the hip joints, ankles, and knees. Many athletes, such as runners and cyclists, find that Pigeon Pose can help maintain a healthy range of movement in the hips. Regular practice leads to a quicker recovery from training and a decreased risk of injury.

## Level

Intermediate

## Benefits

This asana stretches the muscles of the pelvic area, in particular, the gluteal muscles and hip flexors. This leads to improved posture and increases the ability to practise other yoga asanas that require a large range of movement through the hips without causing strain.

## Caution

For those with injuries to the knee, such as damage to the tendons or ligaments, caution should be taken when practising Pigeon Pose.

For those with lower back injuries, such as sciatica or herniated vertebral discs, Pigeon Pose should be modified.

### ⊕ Modifications and props

If the lower back is injured, move into this asana very slowly and support the body by placing a yoga block or folded blanket underneath the right hip.

For knee injuries, place the right foot closer to the hips, so the bent knee is less extended, and place a yoga block or folded blanket underneath the right hip for support.

###  Try to

Lengthen the left leg, so the stretch is felt in the hip flexors of the back leg.

Keep the bodyweight centred to avoid stress on the joints.

Keep the right knee in line with the right side of the pelvis. This will ensure an effective stretch through the gluteal muscles.

###  Try not to

Avoid dropping the heel of the back foot out to the side, and instead stretch the toes back until a stretch is felt across the top of the ankle.

Avoid positioning the right foot forwards to the point where discomfort is felt in the right knee.

# How to do it

**Step 1** ⊘

Begin in Box Pose (p.55).

⊘ **Step 2**

Breathing deeply, transfer more bodyweight into the arms and move the right knee to just behind the right wrist. Now slowly move the right foot over to the left side, so the right lower leg is lying diagonally across the floor. Flex the right ankle so the toes are moving towards the shin; this will help to protect the right knee.

**Step 3** ⊘

Exhale while extending the left leg back, so the left knee joint straightens and the hips move towards the ground. On an inhale, move the hands to either side of the right leg and extend the spine upwards. The shoulders should move down, away from the ears, and the chin should be level with the ground.

⊘ **Step 4**

Exhale and, at the same time, move the upper body forwards, so it is positioned over the front leg, and rest the forearms on the ground in front of the right leg. Keep breathing deeply while the left leg extends back, so the hips sink further towards the ground. Keep the shoulders relaxed and bring the gaze towards the ground in front of the hands.

# Pigeon Pose

## Eka Pada Kapotasana

During Pigeon Pose the right femur is externally rotated to the side and the right knee is in a flexed position, with the lower leg on the ground. This position creates an eccentric lengthening of the quadriceps and gluteus minimus, medius, and maximus, and a concentric contraction of the hamstring. The tibialis anterior concentrically shortens, creating a dorsiflexion at the right ankle, while the soleus lengthens. The left leg is fully extended and the quadriceps shorten concentrically. The hip flexors, in particular, the rectus femoris, lengthen and extend to allow the movement in the hip. The gluteus maximus also concentrically contracts on the left side, helping to extend the hip joint. The spine is in forwards flexion with the quadratus lumborum lengthening eccentrically and the pelvis tilting forwards. Pigeon pose also involves the iliopsoas concentrically shortening on the right side as the upper body moves towards the thigh, and eccentrically lengthening on the left side.

## Anatomy of the pose

**muscle activity**

**prime mover**

1  Quadriceps (left leg)
2  Tibialis anterior (right leg)
3  Hamstrings

**antagonist**

4  Gluteus maximus,
   minimus, and medius
5  Rectus femoris
6  Iliopsoas
7  Quadratus lumborum

(7 beneath thoracolumbar fascia)

**spine**

The spine is in a forwards flexed position in a sagittal plane, moving from a frontal axis.
The pelvis is in an anterior tilt position.

7  Quadratus lumborum
   (beneath thoracolumbar fascia)

4  Gluteus maximus, minimus,
   and medius

Not visible from this view:

6  Iliopsoas (inside hip area, deep)
2  Tibialis anterior (lower leg)

3  Hamstrings

1  Quadriceps

# Wheel Pose

## Urdhva Dhanurasana

Wheel Pose is an advanced asana that is the culmination of proficiency in more basic yoga asanas. Some flexibility of the shoulders, hips, and spine is required to perform it, but the mobility of all these joints is greatly improved with regular practice. The majority of the movement comes from the thoracic region of the spine, which moves into a deep bend, with the back muscles contracting powerfully and shortening. This greatly stretches the abdominal muscles and opens the whole of the upper body, including the front of the ribcage. The arms are fully extended, helping to stretch the shoulder joints and open the chest area. This then allows the spine to move into a deep extension. The feet are positioned hip-width apart and the legs are also extended, stretching the front of the hips, lengthening the hip flexors, and strengthening the quadriceps. The gluteal muscles contract to support the pelvis and lower back. The overall effect is increased flexibility and stability of the shoulders, hips, and spine.

## Level

Advanced

## Benefits

Wheel Pose stretches the entire upper body and increases the range of movement of the spine, shoulders, and hips.

It strengthens the arms and legs, energises the whole body, and is mentally uplifting.

## Caution

Practitioners with back or shoulder injuries or high blood pressure should be cautious when practising Wheel Pose.

### ⊕ Modifications and props

For high blood pressure and more severe back injuries, Shoulder Bridge Pose is a more appropriate asana.

For shoulder injuries, face away from a wall with approximately 0.5 metres space between the wall and the heels. Stretch the arms up overhead and reach the hands back until they can be placed flat onto the wall and the spine arches a little. Practise this modification until the injury heals, before moving into full Wheel Pose.

### ⊘ Try to

Open the chest area by pressing firmly into the hands, extending the elbow joints and allowing the neck to relax.

Work the gluteal muscles without tightening them too much, as this can put undue pressure on the base of the spine.

Keep the elbows in line with the shoulders to ensure maximum support from the triceps.

### ⊗ Try not to

Avoid compressing the lower back; keep the legs firm and lengthen the spine.

Focus on opening the chest by pressing firmly into the hands and gently pushing the chest forwards. This action will help create a more even bend along the spine, as opposed to just bending from the lower back.

# How to do it

**Step 1** ⊙

Begin by lying face up with the legs bent and the feet flat on the ground. Rest the arms by the sides of the body. The breath should be slow and steady.

⊙ **Step 2**

Inhale while placing the hands on the ground either side of the neck, with the fingers pointing towards the shoulders. The elbows should be bent and the whole hands, including the palms and heels, should be in contact with the ground. Stretch out the fingers and thumbs and relax the toes.

**Step 3** ⊙

Now exhale deeply while pressing firmly into the hands and feet, so the legs and arms begin to extend and straighten, lifting the spine and hips from the ground. The front of the ribcage should move upwards, creating an arch in the spine. The knees and elbows should still be partially bent, and the head should be hovering just above the ground.

⊙ **Step 4**

Breathe steadily and fully extend the arms and legs without compressing the lower back. Keep the elbows in line with the shoulders and the knees in line with the ankles. Press firmly into the feet and lift the hips upwards. Relax the gluteal muscles a little and try to relax the upper body, allowing the chest to open and stretch. Relax the neck and head and keep the gaze parallel to the ground, as opposed to looking at the ground.

# Wheel Pose

## Urdhva Dhanurasana

Wheel Pose is an intense backbending position that deeply stretches the chest and abdominal area, and strengthens all the muscles surrounding the spine. The arms are straight and fully extended at the shoulder and elbow joint. The triceps contract concentrically and the deltoids lengthen eccentrically to allow the shoulder joint to open. The muscles of the back, including the erector spinae and latissimus dorsi, concentrically contract powerfully to move the spine into an extended position. The opposing muscle groups, including the pectoral muscles, rectus abdominis, and transversus abdominis, all lengthen eccentrically, allowing the upper body to open and stretch. The hip flexors lengthen eccentrically and the gluteus maximus muscles are in a concentric contraction, extending the hip joint. The knees are in partial flexion due to a concentric contraction of the quadriceps, which work to stabilise the knee joint.

| muscle activity | | |
| --- | --- | --- |
| **prime mover** | 1 Erector spinae<br>2 Latissimus dorsi<br>3 Gluteus maximus<br>4 Quadriceps<br>5 Deltoids | |
| **antagonist** | 6 Rectus abdominis<br>7 Transversus abdominis<br>8 Hip flexors<br>9 Pectoralis major and minor | |

(1 beneath thoracolumbar fascia)

| spine | The spine is in an extended position, moving in a sagittal plane from a frontal axis.<br>The pelvis is in a posterior tilt position. |
| --- | --- |

# Anatomy of the pose

Latissimus dorsi 2

Erector spinae (beneath thoracolumbar fascia) 1

Rectus abdominis 6

Transversus abdominis 7

Hip flexors 8

Gluteus maximus 3

Quadriceps 4

Pectoralis major and minor 9

Deltoids 5

# Cat Pose to Cow Pose

## Marjariasana to Bitilasana

Cat Pose and Cow Pose are gentle asanas that are often performed together (as shown here), and which improve the flexibility of the spine, particularly the thoracic region. During Cat Pose the muscles of the back are stretched while the abdominal muscles are contracted. This action gently massages the abdominal organs. During Cow Pose the muscles of the back contract while the abdominal muscles stretch. By increasing the mobility of the spine in this way, not only are the front and back muscles of the torso both stretched and strengthened, but it is thought that synovial fluid is released to circulate around the vertebrae and blood flow through the muscles, and therefore the spinal discs, is increased.

For both Cat and Cow Pose, the hands are placed with the palms flat to the ground, stretching the wrist flexors. This weight-bearing action gradually increases bone density, and therefore strengthens the wrists. This then makes the wrist flexibility required for asanas such as Wheel Pose more attainable.

## Level

Beginner

## Benefits

Cat and Cow Pose increase the flexibility of the spine, surrounding muscles, and connective tissue, resulting in a decreased likelihood of back pain.

Flexibility and strength of the wrists is also increased.

## Caution

Those with wrist or knee injuries may need to modify this asana.

For neck injuries, including whiplash, maintain neutral alignment of the neck when practising Cow Pose.

 **Modifications and props**

If the knees are injured, a folded blanket can be placed under them for cushioning. If it is not possible to bend the wrists in this way, the arms can be extended, in line with the back, and placed on a chair in front of the head.

### Try to

When moving into Cat Pose, try to create space across the middle of the back by arching from the middle of the spine and drawing the crown of the head and coccyx downwards.

For Cow Pose, elongate from the lower back to the neck and aim for a stretch across the front of the ribcage, while keeping the shoulders down away from the ears.

### Try not to

For Cat Pose, avoid applying a lot of weight to the wrists and instead gently contract the muscles of the torso so that the whole body is working.

When in Cow Pose, avoid overextending the neck and lower back to the point where pressure is felt in these areas. Instead, aim for a sense of length through the neck and lumbar spine, and bend as far as is comfortable.

# How to do it

**Step 1** ⊘

Begin in Box Pose (p.55).

⊙ **Step 2**

To move into Cat Pose, exhale deeply while rounding the spine, moving initially from the centre of the back. The coccyx and crown of the head should point towards the ground, and the chin should move in towards the chest. The scapulae move away from one another, and the abdominal muscles contract and move in towards the spine. The entire back area is lengthened and stretched, and should now be in a concave position.

**Step 3** ⊙

Pause before moving into Cow Pose. Inhale to sink the thoracic spine down as the tail bone and crown of the head move upwards. The shoulders should be drawn down, away from the ears, and the front of the torso should be lengthened from the chin to the navel. The muscles of the back should contract as the front torso muscles lengthen and stretch. The spine should now be in a convex position.

# Cat Pose to Cow Pose

## Marjariasana to Bitilasana

In the starting position for Cat Pose, the triceps concentrically contract to extend the arms, and the iliopsoas muscles shorten and partially flex the hip so the thighs are perpendicular to the ground. During Cat Pose the spine moves into a convex position, which is achieved when the rectus abdominis and transversus abdominis concentrically contract. This leads to a rounding of the thoracic region of the spine, in which the oblique abdominal muscles assist. The pectoral and anterior deltoid muscles also shorten via a concentric contraction to help round the upper back. To allow this articulation of the spine, the erector spinae muscles lengthen eccentrically, and the trapezius muscles stretch to move the scapulae into 'prostration', moving them away from one another. Other muscles of the back that lengthen eccentrically include the splenius capitis, splenius cervicis, and latissimus dorsi.

When moving into Cow Pose, the main muscle groups that lengthen and shorten are effectively reversed to allow the spine to move into a concave position.

NB: The prime movers in Cat Pose become the antagonists when moving into Cow Pose, and vice versa.

| muscle activity | prime mover | **A: CAT POSE**<br>1 Rectus abdominis<br>2 Transversus abdominis<br>3 Internal and external obliques<br>4 Anterior deltoid | **B: COW POSE**<br>1 Erector spinae<br>2 Latissimus dorsi<br>3 Trapezius<br>4 Splenius capitis<br>5 Splenius cervicis<br>6 Longissimus thoracis |
| | antagonist | 5 Erector spinae<br>6 Latissimus dorsi<br>7 Trapezius<br>8 Splenius capitis<br>9 Splenius cervicis<br>10 Longissimus thoracis | 7 Rectus abdominis<br>8 Transversus abdominis<br>9 Internal and external obliques<br>10 Anterior deltoid |

**spine**

The movement of the spine occurs in a sagittal plane and originates from the frontal axis.

In Cat Pose, the spine is in flexion and the pelvis is in a posterior tilt position.

In Cow Pose, the spine is in extension and the pelvis is in an anterior tilt position.

# Anatomy of the pose

6 Latissimus dorsi

10 Longissimus thoracis
(under 6 and 7)

Erector spinae
(under thoracolumbar
fascia) 5

7 Trapezius

8 Splenius capitis

9 Splenius cervicis
(8 and 9 under Trapezius)

4 Anterior deltoid

3 Internal and
external obliques

1 Rectus abdominis

2 Transversus abdominis

**A** Cat Pose

**B** Cow Pose

Erector 1
spinae

Longissimus 6
thoracis

4 Splenius capitis

5 Splenius cervicis
(4 and 5 under
Trapezius)

10 Anterior deltoid

3 Trapezius

2 Latissimus dorsi

9 Internal and
external obliques

7 Rectus abdominis

8 Transversus abdominis

# Inversions

Inversions involve the head being positioned lower than the heart. There are two distinct groups of inversions – one is relatively calming, and includes Shoulder Stand Pose and Downward-facing Dog Pose; the other is more stimulating, and includes Headstand Pose. The latter type can help the practitioner to overcome emotional blocks, such as fear and lack of confidence. The overall effect of any inversion is improved circulation and renewed oxygen to the brain, thus increasing mental concentration and memory.

# Downward-facing Dog Pose

## Adho Mukha Svanasana

Downward-facing Dog Pose is a fundamental pose that is sometimes used as a resting asana in between more challenging poses. The arms are straight with the hands pressed into the ground and the fingers and thumbs spread out with the middle finger pointing directly forwards. This helps minimise pressure in the wrist joint. This action also strengthens the arms and stretches the shoulder joints and chest, while the muscles of the upper back contract to keep the shoulder blades in the correct alignment.

The spine is in a neutral position and there is an emphasis on lengthening the entire spine, from the sacrum to the neck, and on creating space around the ribcage, too. The legs are straight, with the thighs firm, and the calf muscles lengthen as the heels move towards the ground, increasing flexibility in the ankle joints. The pelvis is tilted forwards, so the sitting bones and coccyx move upwards, stretching the backs of the legs even further. This also enables the lower back and gluteal muscles to stretch more, helping to relieve lower back pain.

**Level**

Beginner

**Benefits**

This asana opens the shoulders and lengthens the muscles along the spine.

It stretches the hamstrings and calf muscles and opens the shoulders, improving overall postural alignment.

**Caution**

Practitioners with low blood pressure may find this is affected when Downward-facing Dog Pose is held for extended periods of time.

Those with wrist injuries should be cautious when practising this asana.

⊕ **Modifications and props**

To modify this asana, remain on the knees with the hips aligned over the knees. Extend the arms forwards and sink the chest to the floor, resting the forehead on the ground.

For neck injuries, Downwards-facing Dog Pose can be practised with a yoga block underneath the top of the head to support the neck.

 **Try to**

Lengthen through the spine by pressing firmly into the hands and moving the hips upwards before dropping the heels to the floor and moving the hips back a little.

Relax the neck and move the shoulders away from the head to create space around the neck.

 **Try not to**

Avoid forcing the heels to the floor, as this may strain the Achilles tendon. Instead, aim for a gentle stretch in the shoulder joint by pressing into the hands, and allow the heels to slowly drop towards the ground.

# How to do it

**Step 1** ⊘

Begin in Box Pose (p.55).

⊘ **Step 2**

Move the hands forwards by approximately the length of one hand. Stretch the fingers out, ensuring the middle finger is pointing forwards. Tuck the toes under.

⊘ **Step 3**

Now inhale while pressing firmly into the hands and lifting the knees from the floor, gradually raising the hips upwards. At first, keep the knees slightly bent and the heels lifted away from the ground. Focus on elongating the spine and lifting the sitting bones upwards. Keep pressing firmly into the hands and exhale deeply.

⊘ **Step 4**

Now let the heels drop towards the ground so the knee joints straighten. The arms, spine, and legs should now be straight. Gently contract the abdominal muscles and move the shoulder blades away from the head, keeping the neck relaxed. The gaze should be towards the lower legs. Breathe steadily.

# Downward-facing Dog Pose

## Adho Mukha Svanasana

In Downward-facing Dog Pose, the arms and legs are extended, helping to stretch several major muscle groups, while the quadriceps shorten concentrically to extend the knees. The deltoid muscles lengthen eccentrically to extend the arms from the shoulder joint, and then internally rotate the upper arms, resulting in pronation of the forearms. This internal rotation leads to the stabilisation of the shoulder girdle. There is a concentric contraction of the triceps, allowing the biceps brachii to lengthen eccentrically and the elbow joint to fully extend. The trapezius muscles then contract concentrically to move the scapulae away from the head. The erector spinae is in an eccentric stretch while the iliopsoas shortens concentrically, so the hip joint is only partially flexed. With the pelvis at this angle, the gluteus maximus, hamstrings, soleus, and gastrocnemius all lengthen eccentrically. The ankle joint is in a dorsiflexed position brought about partly by a concentric contraction of tibialis anterior.

**muscle activity**

**prime mover**

| | |
|---|---|
| **1** | Iliopsoas |
| **2** | Quadriceps |
| **3** | Trapezius |
| **4** | Tibialis anterior |
| **5** | Anterior deltoid |

**antagonist**

| | |
|---|---|
| **6** | Hamstrings |
| **7** | Erector spinae |
| **8** | Gluteus maximus |
| **9** | Soleus and gastrocnemius |
| **10** | Posterior deltoid |

(7 beneath thoracolumbar fascia)

**spine**

The spine is in a neutral position, moving in a sagittal plane from a frontal axis.
The pelvis is in an anterior tilt position.

# Anatomy of the pose

**Not visible from this view:**

1  Iliopsoas (inside hip area, deep)

3  Trapezius

7  Erector spinae
   (beneath thoracolumbar fascia)

8  Gluteus maximus

2  Quadriceps

6  Hamstrings

4  Tibialis anterior

Soleus and gastrocnemius  9

5  Anterior deltoid

10  Posterior deltoid

# Shoulder Bridge Pose

## Setu Bandhasana Sarvangasana

Shoulder Bridge Pose is one of the more gentle backbends. It strengthens the legs and back, and increases flexibility in the spine and shoulders. It is a useful asana to practise before more challenging postures such as Wheel Pose, as it stretches the chest and shoulders and mobilises the spine.

The knees are bent with the ankles aligned directly underneath the knees joints and the feet hip-width apart. This position helps to avoid strain on the knee tendons and unnecessary tension in the gluteal muscles. The hips and spine are lifted from the ground until an arch is created through the entire spine. The arms are on the ground under the spine with the hands interlaced, moving the shoulder blades towards one another and the chest towards the chin. This helps to stretch the chest and the front of the shoulders and strengthens the extensor muscles of the spine. The legs work powerfully to keep the knees in alignment with the hips, with the hamstrings and gluteal muscles contracting and the quadriceps lengthening so the knees can bend.

## Level

Intermediate

## Benefits

This asana strengthens the muscles of the spine, legs, and hips.

It increases the flexibility of the chest, shoulders, and spine and invigorates the whole body, increasing energy levels.

## Caution

Practitioners with high blood pressure, or neck or lower back injuries, should be cautious when practising this asana.

### ⊕ Modifications and props

To modify the asana for either high blood pressure or back injuries, support the spine by placing a yoga block or bolster underneath the lower back.

To avoid aggravating neck injuries, do not interlace the fingers under the back. Instead, rest the hands flat on the floor with the arms straight.

### ⊘ Try to

Keep the knees in line with the front hip bones and try to draw the shoulder blades towards one another to create more lift through the chest and spine.

### ⊗ Try not to

Try not to lift the hips to a position where there is pressure on the spine.

Do not allow the knees to be wider apart than the ankles, because this will put strain on the knee joints.

Avoid pressing into the heels and lifting the toes; instead, relax the toes, as this will help to minimise tension in the lower back.

# How to do it

### ⊚ Step 1

Begin by lying face up with the legs bent, feet flat on the floor and hip-width apart.

### Step 2 ⊛

The knees should be aligned directly over the ankles. Rest the arms on the ground either side of the body, with the palms of the hands facing down. Keeping the head and neck still and the feet flat on the ground, exhale as you lift the hips and spine away from the ground. The body should now form a diagonal straight line from the knees to the shoulders, and the spine should be in a neutral position.

### ⊚ Step 3

Now inhale while lifting the pelvis higher, so the chest moves towards the chin and the spine is in a slight backbending position, creating an arch through the middle back. Keep breathing steadily and move the shoulder blades back towards one another while simultaneously moving the arms towards one another. Interlace the fingers underneath the back. Contract the muscles of the lower body, including the gluteal muscles, hamstrings, and lower abdominal muscles.

# Shoulder Bridge Pose

## Setu Bandhasana Sarvangasana

During Shoulder Bridge Pose the hamstrings are concentrically contract, flexing the knees. This creates an eccentric lengthening of the quadriceps and hip flexor muscle groups, which then work as fixators, holding the femurs in place. The gluteus maximus muscles also contract concentrically and supports both the pelvis and sacroiliac joint. The spine, mainly the thoracic region, is in an extended position that is created when the quadratus lumborum and erector spinae muscles contract concentrically. By moving the hips upwards to the full shoulder bridge position, the pectoral and anterior deltoid muscles eccentrically lengthen, and the trapezius muscles contract concentrically to retract the scapulae towards the spine, moving the sternum closer to the chin. The ankle joints are in neutral alignment, with the feet flat to the ground.

## Anatomy of the pose

(2 and 4 beneath thoracolumbar fascia)

2 Erector spinae

4 Quadratus lumborum

6 Hip flexors

5 Trapezius

9 Quadriceps

8 Pectoralis major and minor

7 Deltoids

3 Gluteus maximus

| muscle activity | prime mover | 1 Hamstrings<br>2 Erector spinae<br>3 Gluteus maximus<br>4 Quadratus lumborum<br>5 Trapezius |
| --- | --- | --- |
| | antagonist | 6 Hip flexors<br>7 Deltoids<br>8 Pectoralis major and minor<br>9 Quadriceps |

(2 and 4 beneath thoracolumbar fascia)

**spine**

The spine is in an extended position, moving in a sagittal plane from a frontal axis.
The pelvis is in an anterior tilt position.

1 Hamstrings

# Shoulder Stand Pose

## Sarvangasana

It can take some time before the practitioner is ready for Shoulder Stand Pose, as it requires strength and flexibility of all the major joints. It is an inversion asana (meaning that the head is lower than the heart) and one which strengthens the whole body and improves respiratory function.

The weight of the body is mainly on the shoulders, with the chin tucked in towards the chest, which stretches the neck. The elbows are bent and the hands rest lightly on the middle of the back to support the upper body. The spine lengthens upwards in a straight line, which requires the spinal extensors to stretch and the abdominal muscles to contract to help maintain the position. The legs and feet also stretch upwards and are pressed firmly together. The chest and front of the shoulders are stretched, while the upper back and back of the shoulders contract to move the shoulder blades together. This allows the practitioner to move onto the tops of the shoulders and straighten the spine more effectively.

### Level

Intermediate

### Benefits

Shoulder Stand Pose strengthens the muscles of the back and abdomen and increases the flexibility of the shoulders and spine.

The thyroid gland and abdominal organs are stimulated, improving metabolism. This asana strengths the heart and lungs, which in turn improves respiratory function.

### Caution

Practitioners with neck injuries or high blood pressure should not practise Shoulder Stand Pose.

Those with shoulder or back injuries should practise with caution.

 **Modifications and props**

To modify Shoulder Stand Pose, lie on the back with the knees bent and the soles of the feet against a wall, so the lower legs are parallel to the ground. Push the feet firmly against the wall and lift the hips and spine away from the ground until the knees, hips, and shoulders create one straight line. Place the hands on the back for support, keeping the feet on the wall for additional support.

✓ **Try to**

Reach the feet upwards to create more length through the body and press the legs together firmly, creating a sense of strength though the lower body.

Stretch across the chest area by moving the elbows towards one another. This will also move the bodyweight away from the neck and onto the shoulders.

 **Try not to**

The chin must stay in line with the sternum, so avoid moving the head, as this can injure the neck.

Do not let the weight of the hips rest on the hands; instead, work towards straightening the spine and creating a feeling of lift through the body.

# How to do it

◎ **Step 1**

Begin in Corpse Pose (p.55).

**Step 2** ⌃

Move the arms in towards the sides of the upper body, with the palms of the hands facing down, and press the legs together.

⌃ **Step 3**

Contract the abdominal muscles on an exhale and lift the legs until they are perpendicular to the ground. The hips should remain on the ground and the body should now be at a right angle.

◎ **Step 4**

On an inhale, reach the legs upwards and straighten the spine, so the hips are aligned directly over the shoulders. On an exhale, move the hands closer to the shoulder blades and move the elbows a little closer together. This will help open the front of the shoulders and chest, moving the hips into a more neutral alignment. Reach the feet upwards, stretching all the way to the toes. Ensure the breath is calm and steady.

# Shoulder Stand Pose

## Sarvangasana

During Shoulder Stand Pose the cervical spine is in forwards flexion, while the lumbar and thoracic spine is in a neutral position. The shoulders, pelvis, knees, and ankles are all in alignment. To move the spine into this position, the latissimus dorsi and erector spinae muscles initially stretch eccentrically, then contract concentrically, and finally isometrically to stabilise the upper body. The rectus abdominis also helps to stabilise the upper body, acting as a fixator muscle. The pelvis is in a neutral alignment and the legs are fully extended away from the hips. This position occurs when the gluteus maximus contracts concentrically and the hip flexors lengthen eccentrically. The knees are then fully extended and the quadriceps and hamstrings are in an isometric contraction, fixating the legs in this extended position. The ankle joints plantarflex the feet when the gastrocnemius and soleus shorten via a concentric contraction. To move the arms into the flexed position, the anterior deltoids, pectoral muscles, and triceps all lengthen eccentrically, and the biceps brachii, trapezius, and posterior deltoids all shorten concentrically.

**muscle activity**

**prime mover**

| | |
|---|---|
| **1** | Latissimus dorsi |
| **2** | Quadriceps |
| **3** | Gastrocnemius |
| **4** | Biceps brachii |
| **5** | Gluteus maximus |
| **6** | Deltoids |

**antagonist**

| | |
|---|---|
| **7** | Hamstrings |
| **8** | Erector spinae |
| **9** | Pectoralis major and minor |

(8 beneath thoracolumbar fascia)

**spine**

The thoracic and lumbar areas of the spine are in a neutral position, and the cervical spine is in forwards flexion.
The spine moves in a sagittal plane from a frontal axis.
The pelvis is also in a neutral position.

# Anatomy of the pose

**Not visible from this view:**

8 Erector spinae (on back)

Gastrocnemius 3

Hamstrings 7

2 Quadriceps

Gluteus maximus 5

Latissimus dorsi 1

9 Pectoralis major and minor

6 Deltoids

Biceps brachii 4

# Plough Pose

## Halasana

Plough Pose is an inverted asana, meaning the head is lower than the heart, which increases circulation and invigorates the whole body. It should be practised towards the end of a yoga session, when the body is fully warmed-up and already stretched, so as to avoid injury. It stimulates the thyroid, adrenal, and pituitary glands by compressing the front of the upper body, which helps to balance the metabolic system.

Several major muscle groups are stretched, leading to improved flexibility of the spine, shoulders, and legs. The spinal extensor muscles are lengthened and the muscles of the neck are deeply stretched. The arms are fully straightened, stretching the biceps brachii and the front of the shoulders. The muscles of the upper back, mainly the trapezius, contract to draw the shoulder blades together. This in turn stretches the chest area, helping to improve posture. The legs are straight and the toes are tucked under, which stretches the hamstring and calf muscles.

## Level

Intermediate

## Benefits

The whole spine is stretched in Plough Pose, increasing the flexibility of the upper body.

The compression through the front of the upper body stimulates the thyroid gland and abdominal organs, which in turn stimulates the digestive system.

## Caution

Practitioners with neck injuries or high blood pressure should avoid Plough Pose.

Those with lower back injuries should also practise with caution.

 **Modifications and props**

If the full asana is too intense, keep the hands on the middle of the back and rest the feet on a bolster or some yoga blocks, so the stretch of the spine is lessened.

⊙ **Try to**

Create space in the upper body by lengthening the spine.

Move the shoulder blades towards one another by stretching the arms away from the body, increasing the stretch across the chest and front of the shoulders.

Always keep the head and neck still in Plough Pose to avoid injury.

 **Try not to**

Avoid rounding the spine and instead straighten the back by moving the hips upwards, creating a straight line from the shoulders to the hips.

Let the chin move towards the chest but avoid placing undue strain on the neck. If the neck is uncomfortable, slowly move out of the asana and rest.

# How to do it

**⊲ Step 1**

Begin in Corpse Pose (p.55).

**Step 2 ⊳**

Move the arms in towards the sides of the upper body, with the palms of the hands facing down, and press the legs together. On an exhale, contract the abdominal muscles and lift the legs until they are perpendicular to the ground. The hips should remain on the ground and the body should now be at a right angle.

**⊼ Step 3**

Press firmly into the hands and inhale while lifting the hips and spine from the floor. Breathe evenly and move slowly until the spine is straightened, with the hips aligned over the shoulders. The legs should now be parallel to the floor. Bend the elbows and place the hands on the middle of the back to support the upper body.

**⊽ Step 4**

With the legs straight, bring the feet to the ground and tuck the toes under so the heels are aligned over the balls of the feet. Contract the thigh muscles and now bring the arms down to rest straight out on the ground. On an exhale, stretch the front of the shoulders by interlacing the hands and fully extending the arms.

# Plough Pose

## Halasana

In Plough Pose the major muscle groups of the back, the erector spinae and latissimus dorsi, lengthen eccentrically, while the hip flexors, mainly the iliopsoas, contract concentrically to move the legs towards the torso. The gluteus maximus also stretches eccentrically to increase the angle at the back of the pelvis. This action moves the spine into a neutral position and the hips into a partially flexed position. The triceps contract concentrically and the arms are fully extended with the forearms pronated. This results in an eccentric stretch of the pectoral muscles and anterior deltoids, and a concentric contraction of the posterior deltoids and trapezius muscles. The hamstrings are eccentrically lengthened and the quadriceps are concentrically contracted, which fully extends the knee joints. The ankles are in dorsiflexion, stretching the soleus and gastrocnemius muscles. The neck is in forwards flexion.

## Anatomy of the pose

8  Gluteus maximus

Quadriceps  2

Latissimus dorsi  7

Erector spinae
(beneath thoracolumbar fascia)  5

Deltoids  4

Triceps  3

## muscle activity

### prime mover

1  Iliopsoas
2  Quadriceps
3  Triceps
4  Deltoids

### antagonist

5  Erector spinae
6  Hamstrings
7  Latissimus dorsi
8  Gluteus maximus

(5 beneath thoracolumbar fascia)

### spine

The lumbar and thoracic spine regions should be in a neutral position and the cervical spine in forwards flexion. The spine moves in a sagittal plane from a frontal axis. The pelvis is in a slight posterior tilt.

6  Hamstrings

Not visible from this view:

1  Iliopsoas (inside hip area, deep)

# Headstand Pose

## Shirshasana

Headstand Pose is one of the more challenging inversions within the yoga system and has many benefits. By inverting the body in this way, blood flows to the brain, while gravity stimulates the blood's return in the veins, improving overall circulation. The respiratory rate is also increased, which helps to strengthen the lungs, improving overall well-being.

All the major muscle groups work hard to stabilise the body and maintain balance. The arms are bent with the fingers and thumbs interlaced, while the muscles across the upper back move the shoulder blades away from the head and neck. This creates a strong framework for the head and neck area. The core muscles, namely the rectus and transversus abdominis, and the lower back muscles help to fix the spine in place. The legs are fully extended from the hips, with the gluteal and hip flexor muscles supporting the pelvis. The legs are pressed together firmly with the feet stretching upwards, giving the sense of strength and lift through the whole body.

### Level

Advanced

### Benefits

This asana is invigorating and rejuvenating. It strengthens the shoulders and upper back muscles in particular, as well as greatly improving core stability.

Regular practice of Headstand Pose also helps to build self-confidence.

### Caution

Those with high blood pressure, or neck or shoulder injuries, should not practise Headstand Pose.

### ⊕ Modifications and props

To modify this asana, remain at stage three and practise aligning the hips over the shoulders. When ready to move up into a full headstand, a wall can be used for support (facing away from the wall), while getting used to lifting the legs.

### ⊘ Try to

Create space for the neck by staying strong across the upper back and pressing the forearms into the ground.

From the legs, imagine the feet are being gently pulled upwards, creating a sense of lift through the entire body.

Keep the spine in a neutral position by flattening the lower back area so the front of the ribcage draws in, as though moving in towards the middle spine.

### ⊗ Try not to

Avoid resting on the head; instead, contract the trapezius muscles, so the upper back and shoulder joints create support for the head and neck.

Avoid arching the lower back area, as this puts pressure on the vertebral discs.

Never move the head or neck while in this position, as injury may occur.

# How to do it

### ⌄ Step 1

Begin in Box Pose (p.55).

### ⌃ Step 2

Place the forearms on the ground, keeping the elbows shoulder-width apart. Now interlace the fingers and thumbs tightly and press the little-finger edges of the hands firmly onto the ground. The palms of the hands should not be pressed together. Move the knees approximately 20 centimetres closer to the arms, and place the back of the head into the palms of the hands, resting the crown of the head lightly on the ground. The spine should be rounded at this point.

### Step 3 ⊙

Tuck the toes under and, with the feet still on the ground, exhale and straighten the legs. Move the feet closer to the upper body until the hips are aligned directly over the shoulders. The spine should now be straight. Now move the shoulders away from the head by working the upper back and shoulder muscles. There should be no pressure on the head or tension in the neck. Keep the shoulders strong and the breath steady.

### ◁ Step 4

Contract the abdominal muscles and, on an inhale, lift the feet from the floor, bending the knees. Move the feet towards the buttocks. Keep the thighs close to the abdomen and the hips stacked over the shoulders so the spine remains straight.

### Step 5 ⊙

Slowly exhale while reaching the feet directly upwards until the legs are completely straight. The body should now be in one straight line. Lengthen through the whole body and avoid arching the lower back. Contract the abdominal muscles firmly to support the spine, and keep the shoulder joints active and the chin parallel to the ground to avoid tension in the neck. Keep breathing steadily throughout.

# Headstand Pose

## Shirshasana

During Headstand Pose there is equal length through the front and back of the upper body, as it is in a neutral alignment, and the rectus abdominis and latissimus dorsi work to fixate the spine in this position. The elbows flex as the biceps brachii shorten and the triceps lengthen. The deltoids are in a concentric contraction and work in synergy with the rotator cuff muscle groups. The upper and lower trapezius and rhomboid muscles contract to depress and then retract the scapulae, creating support for the cervical spine. The gluteus maximus muscles contract concentrically to extend the legs away from the pelvis, while the hip flexors, including the iliopsoas muscles, stabilise the hips. The quadriceps shorten concentrically, extending the knee joints, and the adductor muscles press the legs together. The feet are plantarflexed and the tibialis anterior is lengthened eccentrically.

**muscle activity**

**prime mover**

1 Gluteus maximus
2 Biceps brachii
3 Deltoids
4 Trapezius
5 Rhomboids
6 Adductors
7 Quadriceps

**antagonist**

8 Rectus abdominis
9 Latissimus dorsi

(5 beneath trapezius)

**spine**

The spine is in a neutral position and therefore does not move within a plane.
The pelvis is also in a neutral position.

# Anatomy of the pose

**Not visible from this view:**

6   Adductors (inner thigh)

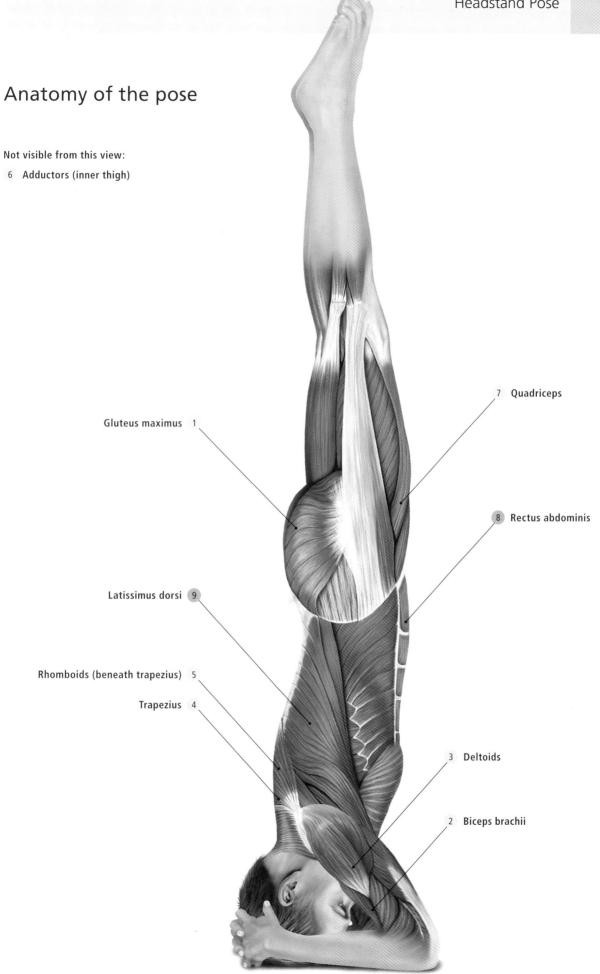

7   Quadriceps

Gluteus maximus   1

8   Rectus abdominis

Latissimus dorsi   9

Rhomboids (beneath trapezius)   5

Trapezius   4

3   Deltoids

2   Biceps brachii

# Sequences

Yoga asanas can be linked together to form different yoga sequences. Variations of these sequences give us the many different styles of hatha yoga there are today. The classic Sun Salutation sequence is a good place to start when building up a practice of a yoga sequence, and there are many styles and levels of Sun Salutation to choose from. The following is taken from ashtanga yoga.

The first version is a modified version of the original ashtanga yoga Sun Salutation A, also known as Surya Namaskara A. This is generally repeated five times before moving on to another yoga sequence.

**Modified Sun Salutation:**

**Step 1**

Begin in Mountain Pose (p.54).

Inhale, reach the arms up overhead, and lift the gaze towards the hands.

**Step 2**

Exhale and fold forwards into Standing Forward Bend (p.110).

Inhale and extend the spine away from the thighs, with the fingertips on the ground.

**Step 3**

Exhale and step the feet back into High Plank Pose (Kumbhakasana).

Inhale and rest the knees on the ground. Exhale and lower the upper body to the ground, so the body is now flat on the ground.

**Step 4**

Inhale and lift the upper spine into Cobra Pose (p.142).

**Step 5**

Exhale and move into Box Pose (p.55).

**Step 6**

Tuck the toes under and lift into Downward-facing Dog Pose (p.164).

**Step 7**

Step the feet forwards into Standing Forward Bend (p.110).

**Step 8**

Inhale and lift the upper body to standing, reaching the arms overhead. On an exhale, rest them by the sides of the body in Mountain Pose (p.54).

**Traditional Sun Salutation:**

### Step 1

Begin in Mountain Pose (p.54).

Inhale, reach the arms up overhead, and lift the gaze towards the hands.

### Step 2

Exhale and fold forwards into Standing Forward Bend (p.110).

Inhale and extend the spine away from the thighs, with the fingertips on the ground.

### Step 3

Exhale and jump the feet back into High Plank Pose (Kumbhakasana).

### Step 4

Keep exhaling and lower the body to Four-limbed Staff Pose (Chaturanga).

### Step 5

Inhale and lift the upper spine into Upward-facing Dog Pose (p.146).

### Step 6

Exhale, tuck the toes under, and lift into Downward-facing Dog Pose (p.164).

### Step 7

Inhale and jump the feet forwards. On an exhale, fold into Standing Forward Bend (p.110) .

### Step 8

Inhale and lift the upper body to standing, reaching the arms overhead. On an exhale, rest them by the sides of the body in Mountain Pose (p.54).

## Hip-opening Sequence

By incorporating carefully selected asanas, sequences can be tailored to create different outcomes and to work particular areas of the body. For example, a sequence that is focused on opening and stretching the hips would incorporate several asanas that gently stretch the quadriceps, adductors, hip flexors, and gluteal muscles. These movements could prepare the hips for a deeper stretch, such as Cobbler's Pose (p.136) or Pigeon Pose (p.150), and would help reduce the risk of injury.

The following example shows how asanas could be linked into a hip-opening sequence:

**1. Triangle Pose** (p.62)

**2. Warrior I Pose** (p.70)

**3. Dancer's Pose** (p.96)

**4. Standing Forward Bend** (p.110)

**5. Half Lord of the Fishes Pose** (p.132)

**6. Seated Forward Bend** (p.124)

**7. Cobbler's Pose** (p.136)

**8. Pigeon Pose** (p.150)

**9. Downward-facing Dog Pose** (p.164)

**10. Corpse Pose** (p.55)

## Energising Sequence

Sequences can also be assembled to challenge the body, for example, by incorporating asanas that move the spine into an extended position, such as in Wheel Pose. This invigorates the body and increases energy levels, partly because backbends release adrenaline, and so work well if the person wishes to stimulate the body and mind. An example of this kind of sequence is as follows:

**1. Cat Pose** (p.158)

**2. Cow Pose** (p.158)

**3. Chair Pose** (p.58)

**4. Dancer's Pose** (p.96)

**5. Standing Forward Bend** (p.110)

**6. Cobra Pose** (p.142)

**7. Downward-facing Dog Pose** (p.164)

**8. Upward-facing Dog Pose** (p.146)

**9. Downward-facing Dog Pose** (p.164)

**10. Wheel Pose** (p.154)

**11. Shoulder Bridge Pose** (p.168)

**12. Corpse Pose** (p.55)

# Glossary

**Abduction** Movement of a limb away from the midline of the body.

**Adduction** Movement of a limb towards the midline of the body.

**Antagonist** A muscle that relaxes and lengthens while another, the 'agonist', contracts.

**Asana** A posture adopted during the practice of hatha yoga that brings about increased well-being.

**Cartilaginous joint** A slightly movable joint in which cartilage joins bones together.

**Chakra** The seven centres of energy within the body that align with areas of the spine.

**Circumduction** A circular movement of a limb extending from the joint at which the movement originates. Full circumduction allows for 360-degree movement.

**Concentric contraction** A type of muscle activity that results in the muscle contracting, or shortening, such as when a weight is lifted.

**Depression** Movement in a downwards (inferior) direction, such as the shoulders moving down away from the head.

**Dorsiflexion** A type of movement (of the ankle or wrist) that causes the toes/fingers to move up towards the front of the ankle/wrist.

**Eccentric contraction** A type of muscle activity that results in the muscle lengthening, such as when a weight is lowered through a range of motion.

**Elevation** Movement in an upwards (superior) direction, such as a shoulder shrug, during which the shoulders lift towards the head.

**Extension** A movement that increases the angle between two body parts. Extension at the elbow increases the angle between the upper arm and the forearm.

**Fibrous joint** A form of articulation in which the bones are connected by a fibrous tissue, mainly collagen.

**Fixator** A muscle that acts as a stabiliser of the body during movement of another part.

**Flexion** A movement that decreases the angle between two body parts. Flexion at the elbow decreases the angle between the upper arm and the forearm.

**Frontal plane** An imaginary vertical plane dividing the body into anterior (front) and posterior (back) portions.

**Hatha yoga** The system of yoga in which asanas are practised for increased well-being.

**Inversion** A yoga asana in which the head is positioned lower than the heart.

**Isometric contraction** A type of muscle activity that results in no change in the length of the muscle, such as when pushing against an immovable object.

**Lever** A rigid structure that moves around an axis point when force is applied. For example, an arm is a lever and its axis point is the shoulder joint.

**Planes of movement** Used to describe movements of the body, referring to imaginary 'planes' that divide the body into sections.

**Plantarflexion** The movement in which the toes and foot point away from the body, so the angle between the foot and back of the leg is decreased.

**Pranayama** The practice of controlled breathing techniques used in yoga.

**Prime mover** A muscle that contracts to produce a movement. Also known as an **agonist**.

**Range of movement** The measurement of movement, measured in degrees, around a specific joint or body part.

**Sagittal plane** An imaginary vertical line running front to back, dividing the body into right and left. Also known as the **lateral plane**.

**Synergist** A muscle that assists other muscles to accomplish a movement.

**Synovial joint** A freely movable joint in which bony surfaces are covered by articular cartilage and are connected by a fibrous connective-tissue capsule lined with a synovial membrane.

**Transverse plane** An imaginary plane that divides the body into superior (upper) and inferior (lower) sections. Also known as the **horizontal** or **axial plane**.

# Index